The Way to Be Healthier, Happier, and Live Longer!

Here's an integrated program of jogging, aerobics, and diet that will enable you to achieve new levels of physical fitness, mental keenness, and emotional stability.

This plan is as natural as breathing: aerobics is a method of expanded oxygen consumption within the body, and jogging is its most effective practice. Aerobic exercise, combined with a diet patterned on your individual needs, can win you improved appearance, weight and appetite control, and a less stressful, healthier life.

Roy Ald was prompted to write this guide by his concern over national health statistics: here is the first book to incorporate the three basics essential to keeping fit—jogging, aerobics, diet, and a special dividend of delicious non-fattening recipes!

Other SIGNET Books of Special Interest

Jogging, Aerobics & Diet

ONE IS NOT ENOUGH— YOU NEED ALL THREE

By Roy Ald

With a Foreword by
M. THOMAS WOODALL, PH.D.
Director of Physical Education
Research Laboratory
Eastern Illinois University

A SIGNET BOOK
NEW AMERICAN LIBRARY
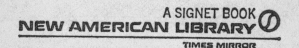
TIMES MIRROR

SIGNET TRADEMARK REG. U.S. PAT. OFF. AND FOREIGN COUNTRIES
REGISTERED TRADEMARK—MARCA REGISTRADA
HECHO EN CHICAGO, U.S.A.

SIGNET, SIGNET CLASSICS, MENTOR, PLUME AND MERIDIAN BOOKS
are published by The New American Library, Inc.,
1301 Avenue of the Americas, New York, New York 10019

FIRST SIGNET PRINTING, DECEMBER, 1968

7 8 9 10 11 12 13 14 15

PRINTED IN THE UNITED STATES OF AMERICA

CONTENTS

FOREWORD, *by M. Thomas Woodall, Ph.D.*   *ix*

INTRODUCTION   *xi*

PART I / *AEROBIC FITNESS*

The Exercise Dropout   *17*

The Breath of Life   *19*

The Vital Balance   *22*

Enter Mr. Machine   *23*

The Age Trap   *25*

RXercise   *29*

Pinpointing Your Exercise Needs   *31*

The Many Faces of Fatigue   *34*

Aerobic and Other Exercises   *37*

Run for Your Life and Health   *41*

The Heart of the Matter   *43*

The Fallacy of the Gung-Ho Runner   *45*

The Aerobic Runner's Creed   *47*

The Rhyme and Reason of Your Body Rhythm   *49*

The Running Steps to Aerobic Fitness   *54*

The Self-Pacing Method   *55*

PART II / *THE AEROBIC RUNNING PROGRAM*

Aerobic Fitness in Action   *61*

The Aerobic Runner's Ten Commandments of Fitness   *62*

The *Right* Running Schedule for You   *63*

The Harvard Step Test

On the Importance of Preconditioning   *66*

Training the Heart Muscle   67
The Aerobic Runner's Preconditioning Exercise Section   70
   Where It All Began
   Bridging the Activity Gap
The Aerobic Support Exercises: Supplesthenics   72
Time Training   75
Preconditioning/Basic Shape-up Plan   77
Preconditioning/Intermediate Shape-up Plan   85
Preconditioning/Advanced Shape-up Plan   88
Basic Time-Trainer Running Plans   90
   Run the Milestone
Intermediate Time-Trainer Running Plans   102
   Run the Milestone
Advanced Time-Trainer Running Plans   117
Clothing and Climate   123
Women in the Running   125
Running from Illness   127
Running as Therapeutic Treatment   130
The Fat Cycle   132

PART III / *THE AEROBIC ENERGY-
   CONTROL DIET*

The Candidates for Diet and Fitness   135
Food Energy and Exercise Energy   136
The Energy Food   138
Setting the Record Straight   140
Special E/C Diet Sections   142
The Diet for All "Plussers"   143
Control Your Weight Loss   144
How to Use the E/C Reducing Diet   146
Your Eating Habitracker   147
   Eating Habitracker Profile
Energy-Control Diet Planner   156
Energy-Control Breakfast Menus   158
Energy-Control Mealmaker Menus   161
vi

Energy-Control Mealmaker Recipes   164
Energy-Control Family Fitness Recipes   169
Salads: An Energy-Control Support Food   174
Soup: An E/C Diet Support Food   179
Appetite Snack Supports   188
Desirable Weight Scale   190

MY LIFELONG EDUCATION and special area of study and research has been the human body. And if I were asked to advise man or woman in regard to those few absolute essentials owed their bodies to maintain health, vitality, and general well-being, I would tell them—"Run for Your Life."

It is the same counsel which I give those members of the running group which I conduct as the Run for Your Life Program, among them medical doctors, bankers, lawyers, ministers, salesmen and businessmen. They are of *all* ages, the oldest in his seventies. Obviously, I do not consider age a deterrent in a running or jogging program. I have expressed opinions in this regard, correspondent to Roy Ald's in his section "The Age Trap." All individuals will show different limitations as they participate in a jogging program, but my own experience has demonstrated that, of these differences, chronological age is of lesser importance and that it is very possible to be physiologically many years younger than the chronological age.

Roy Ald's running program is especially discerning in that it emphasizes "the whole human being" and the relationship of the psychological to the physical benefits of vigorous aerobic exercise. In the stressful, highly mechanized world in which we live, inactivity, obesity, and hypertension have been implicated in heart disease, as well as the other high mortality diseases. And this exercise program directed toward the alleviation of these problems makes a worthwhile contribution.

I applaud this same completeness of approach in the author's handling of exercise and diet—as opposite halves of a single system. Exercise of itself cannot solve the overweight problem, as diet alone cannot bring physical fitness. The underlying principle of Roy Ald's Energy-Control Diet, which is based upon a reasonable reduction of the energy foods, and his abhorrence of crash diets are views which I have expressed in my own Run for Your Life program and booklet.

In all of these respects and the many others, such as the emphasis in a running program of *endurance* and not speed, of rhythmic pacing, of heart training, the recommendation of three workout periods per week, I find this book an eminently sensible one. I urge all those who would wish to profit by its wisdom to begin a jogging program without delay.

Philosopher John Locke said, "A sound mind in a sound

body is a short but full description of a happy state in this world. He that has these two has little more to wish for, and he that wants either of them, will be but little the better for anything else."

And to those who nod in agreement and *intend* to pursue this worthy objective when they have the "time", I would add—there are 336 half-hour periods in each seven-day week. Are you so busy that you can't part with three of them? If so, then as a sedentary adult, you are "too busy." Consider for a moment your weekly responsibilities. As a sedentary adult, the physical activity related to your job is practically nil. The numerous committee and other meetings, along with social, service, fraternal, religious, musical, and other group obligations, provide circulorespiratory benefits only on rare occasions. Truly, our society has us caught up in a whirlwind of activity, but none of it is physical.

We are deteriorating and dying from C.H.D.,* not low I.Q. Make the time to care for your body and live a *quality* life!

M. THOMAS WOODALL, PH.D.
Director of Physical Education
Research Laboratory,
Eastern Illinois University,
Charleston, Illinois

*C. H. D.: Coronary Heart Disease.

INTRODUCTION

THIS BOOK offers to the reader what Dr. Warren Guild, Associate in Medicine at Harvard University and President of the American College of Sports Medicine, has called "living insurance." Whether you are a man or a woman, twenty-five, fifty-five, or seventy-five, aerobic jogging exercises can help you extend your lifespan and add new vitality to each day lived. It can show you the way to an improved, younger appearance, weight and appetite control, and a happier, less stressful existence.

Jogging programs similar to the one conducted by San Diego State College's Dr. Frederick W. Kasch, Director of Physical Education, and Associate Director John L. Boyer, M.D., commonly include among the participants cardiac patients, diabetics, sufferers from high blood pressure, asthma, and other ailments. This prescription of running in preventative and therapeutic medicine is a practice widely supported by prominent medical specialists, such as Dr. Wilhelm Rabb, organizer of the Stowe, Vermont, Conference on Preventative Cardiology, Dr. Carlton B. Chapman, past president of the American Heart Association, and Dr. Myrvin Ellestad, Director of Cardio Pulmonary Laboratory at Memorial Hospital, Long Beach, California, each of whom is a confirmed jogger. Dr. Rabb, at seventy-two, runs at home daily and recommends running "as the best of all physical exercises." Dr. Guild, who is also a U.S. Presidential consultant on physical fitness, runs five to eight miles daily, as Dr. Chapman has been doing for the past 13 years. Recognition and data confirming the salutary effects of running have been forthcoming from England, Sweden, Japan, Russia, Australia, and New Zealand. Dr. Rabb insists that "older persons are capable of both beginning and conducting a strict program," and in his opinion, "Millions should be doing it."

For one deeply involved in physical fitness for the past 26 years as a writer, lecturer, marathon runner, and instructor of running groups, this recognition of the virtues of running and jogging has been long overdue. Only a few brief years ago, I had to scan the newspapers to find a line or two on the subject, which was confined strictly to the sports page. Now, almost daily, I am besieged with articles in national magazines, with photographs of jogging celebrities, the likes of Mayor John V. Lindsay of New York City, Evangelist Billy Graham, Senator

William Proxmire, movie personalities Tony Curtis and Mitzi Gaynor, and Governor George Romney of Michigan. Insofar as the publicity serves to amplify the important message "Run for Your Life and Health," I thoroughly approve of it. But not without some reservations. One of them is the concern that the subject will be treated as a passing fad, with exercise books dealing in part with fact and fancy, wild claims, and injudicious running instructions that may permanently lead away from the activity those who are most in need of reinvigorating and restorative effects. It is this concern which has spurred me to this task of authorship.

Jogging, Aerobics & Diet is a unique exercise book and, in several respects, a revolutionary one. It will place in your hands the medically proven aerobic oxygen-revitalizing benefits of running as a life-giving activity. But it will not stop there. It will help you and millions of other Americans to recognize their highly individual need for exercise and equip you to overcome the common resistance to exercise on a regular and continuing basis. It is not enough to say that at last the medical profession and physical educators have found running to be a potential breakthrough in many critical areas in the field of public health. With all due respects to the potential, it cannot be realized unless the characteristic known to professionals as "the exercise barrier" is overcome. It is useless and a blow to the exerciser's self-esteem to prod and deride him as "a quitter" or conjure up the old bogey, "weak willpower." There is no legitimate basis whatever for such a thing as willpower, either in medicine or the science of human behavior. What is being interpreted as a failure on the part of the individual is really a failure of such exercise programs.

Jogging, Aerobics & Diet IS THE FIRST EXERCISE SYSTEM TO TREAT THE RELUCTANCE TO EXERCISE AS A SYMPTOM OF THE BODY'S WEAKENED AEROBIC CONDITION. It demonstrates how running may be used to overcome this universal barrier to renewed vigor and buoyant spirits. And in doing so, it reveals the relationship of aerobic running to the three dimensions of the human system—physical, mental, and emotional. It hands over to the exerciser a method of self-control with which he or she can break the cycle of damaging stress and hypertension which is the trigger for the primary diseases of Western civilization. These very same ailments, previously enumerated, respond well to sustained running programs. Dr. Heinze Lehmann, Professor of Psychiatry at McGill University, stated before the symposium on The Emotional Basis of Illness that "In the Western world of today, stresses, tensions and emotional onslaughts seem to have replaced hunger and infection, the great hazards of yesterday." A report from Moscow announced that heart disease was the number one killer in the Soviet Union and that more and more Russians, like American citizens, were dying of cardiovascular and related diseases brought on by worry and general nervousness.

The recognition of this crucial physical-emotional relationship can help extend the benefits of aerobic running to millions of Americans who are entirely unaware of their urgent need for it. Those faced with continuous levels of anxiety about money, job security, and emotionally strained relationships need to run to dilate constricted arteries. There are the frustrated, restless types for whom running will provide a pent-up release of nervous energies; and the academic think-tank mental types; the accountants, attorneys, those whose work is largely cerebral. For them, the remark of famous heart surgeon Dr. Paul Dudley White is apropos: "There is more truth than humor in the saying that if you want to know how flabby your brain is, feel your leg muscles."

As a physical therapist, I had long ago learned to interpret these characteristics as signs of the body's need for vigorous aerobic, "air-taking" exercise. Prompt action could disrupt the debilitating cycle before there was lasting damage. Every movement, thought, and feeling is accompanied by gland and nerve function. When depressed, the intake of oxygen is reduced and the circulation slowed. There is less energy for the muscles, and fatigue sets in to further reduce activity. There is a depressed organ function and the weakening performance of an underexercised heart. The sluggish, inactive body uses food differently, leading to the overweight condition . . . leading to even *less* physical activity.

The first duty of an aerobic running system, as I see it, is to train the person to recognize these conditions as "exercise signs." The second is to prepare him to fulfill these highly individualized needs. This means that the exercise system has to take into account those factors which determine what I call "individual runability": general health and the attitude toward the running exercises; bodyweight and eating habits; the period of prior inactivity, heart condition, and exercise limits, as well as the individual's pacing and body rhythms.

This seems like a rather tall order indeed, compared to those running programs which are little more than a collection of contests racing against time and distance. They urge the exerciser to keep up a breakneck pace, to cram the exercise to save three or four minutes! grading him as well, very poor, poor, fair, and so on, according to his showing.

Is it any wonder that this life-giving and lifesaving activity is performed by so few of those who need it the most? And that among those who *do* venture, so many do not keep up their good intentions. In an activity so vital to health and well-being, it is a sad loss.

It need be no longer.

Jogging, Aerobics & Diet is a highly individualized exercise system. All of the points essential for a realization of the full benefits of aerobic running are built into the system and the exercise schedules. Running becomes an easier, freer, more natural physical release with the Self-Pacing Method and the practice of Time Training. The system for advancing the exercise limit is even more precise.

With all of this, and requiring incomparably *less* attention to detail, the runner is given control over the advancement of his capacities and his heart function. In this regard, the exerciser will find the Heart-Training technique, adapted from Dr. Frederick W. Kasch's findings, of inestimable value. And finally, with the Aerobic Energy-Control Diet as a complement to the Aerobic Fitness Schedules, the runner comes to recognize and to treat *overweight* and *underexercise* as inseparable parts of a single problem—an insight which gives him new hope for *permanent* weight control.

If the reader assumes from all of the foregoing that *Jogging, Aerobics & Diet* is another one of those new-lease-on-life books, I will not try to dissuade him. A slight distinction should be made, however. This book works! And if the reader would be shown, like that legendary gentleman from Missouri, my suggestion is that he—*run*, not walk, for the nearest exit and start jogging under an open expanse of sky for the freest and most exhiliarating experience of his life. And keep in mind, it is something the doctor ordered. He's even out there hightailing it in pursuit of his own prescription.

ROY ALD

PART 1

Aerobic Fitness

The Exercise Dropout

WHILE WRITING THIS BOOK, I had occasion to talk to physiologist Tom Woodall of Eastern Illinois University, who has been studying the effects of running with various groups of joggers over a period of nine years. He strongly emphasized the problem of motivation, what I refer to with my own groups as Get-Up-and-Go Power. There used to be a time when I resorted to what is popularly known among the coaches and athletic instructors as The Pep Talk to instill new runners with the incentive to keep on jogging along. Judging by the number of backsliders, particularly among those who desperately needed the exercise, it was not too successful. For those, like myself, involved in exercise or physical therapy, who recognize the truly life-giving benefits of proper exercise, such dropouts can be discouraging. It was one such experience which supplied me with the way to reduce such dropouts to a bare minimum.

Mr. R. N., a successful civil engineer, fifty-eight years of age and looking ten years older, stepped out during a workout and quietly announced to me that he'd had it. "The life that I live requires hardly any physical effort at all. What's the point of trying to increase my physical capacities if I'm not called upon to use them anyway?" There are a great many reasonable answers to his question. I had used them many times without much success. My father, who ideally combined the characteristics of scholar and athlete, used to tell my brothers and myself on occasions when the remark was called for, "If you *won't* do, then presently you will discover that you *can't* do." Much later, I found the same idea in the writings of the great American psychologist William James, when he wrote, ". . . if we often flinch from making an effort, before we know it, the effort-making capacity is gone. . . . Keep the faculties of effort alive in you by a little gratuitous exercise every day."

Why, I thought, as I faced this successful, mature, and intelligent man, were these thoughts less convincing to him than they were to me? It was then that I realized I was applying them to the capabilities of the human body with a professional understanding of its inner processes. He did not have such a background. For him, the words were a rather shopworn maxim. From my point of view, they gave me a sharp mental picture of the revitalizing effect of aerobic running inside his body.

It was then that I realized that too much was expected of the exerciser or the prospective exerciser. He or she was supposed to put out the effort and do the running and simply take for granted that it was good for practically everything that ailed him. The whole thing seemed farfetched. He'd always associated running as an activity for youngsters and trained athletes, one that put a "strain" on the heart. And it seemed a contradiction to be told, when he was feeling really tired, that he needed to go running! More specifically, it had to be *aerobic* running. He had heard or read about the subject and knew vaguely that it had something to do with getting his body to use more oxygen. If anything, this only added to the confusion. There were just too many loose ends to the whole idea. It was possible to get caught up in the first wave of a fad, the early novelty of which did not last very long. Then the old couch and TV set became a whole lot more appealing than a sweat suit and the honest-to-God sweat that went with it!

These were the thoughts which led me to a new approach in orienting each new group of runners. It was my intention to do something a lot more important than explain details about how the body processes functioned. Quite understandably, this kind of information would be forgotten in a matter of weeks. What I had to do was to imprint upon the mind of each exerciser as vivid a *mental picture* as I had. They had to *see* and be as aware of what aerobic running was doing inside them as they could *see* the movement of their arms and legs as they went along.

"Here is the picture," as I say to my new groups of runners and runnerettes. "Get ready to be imprinted."

The Breath of Life

WHEN WE WISH to distinguish a living thing from an unliving one, we call it *animate*, meaning that it is filled with air or breath. This is the vital force which energizes and moves it. *If suddenly it is relieved of air, it expires.* In order to remain alive, it must consume air, and all animals consume life-giving oxygen. Respiration, breathing in and out, is really the measure of being alive. Since it is oxygen that Man and all living creatures have in common, this is where the word "aerobic" comes in. It means "oxygen-consuming."

Our bodies and those of all living creatures have really been formed as oxygen-burning machines which work in this way:

First Step: "Get that oxygen!"

The oxygen has to be *captured* and brought into the body. The respiratory system does this— mainly the diaphragm and the lungs, the "air bags."

Second Step: "Pass the oxygen around inside!"

The oxygen has to be circulated all over the system, and it is the circulatory system that gets it there, through the veins, arteries, and capillaries, with the powerful heart pump driving it into the blood stream.

Third Step: "Use the oxygen to burn up the food for energy!"

The digestive system helps to process the oxygen, using it to burn the food into energy to power the muscles that keep the body processes going.

The nervous system controls the entire operation. A very neat one and a mighty efficient one—providing that *you* deliver the oxygen to do the job in the first place!

The oxygen is the igniter, the vital spark that fires up the engine. We can manage to get along without food for several weeks, but we'd only last a matter of minutes without oxygen— less than that, if you consider that the brain can be permanently damaged by depriving it of oxygen for four seconds! The thoughts and the emotions—all that makes up the human personality—hangs by a hairbreadth. The most brilliant mind confined to a stuffy room without an adequate oxygen supply is soon reduced to a moronic apathy; the emotions pay the penalty with rapid depression and melancholy; while a rich oxygen supply brings on a state of buoyant vigor and health.

One of my runners, an English literature instructor who has run away from his emphysema from years of excessive smoking, has come up with this bon mot:

PERSPIRATION . . . —which means, literally, breathing
everywhere, as through the skin,
when running vigorously—Brings

INSPIRATION . . . to draw air into the lungs and
"inspirit" with feelings of
courage, cheerfulness, and hope.
Or, the choice of inactivity,
which depresses the spirit, lets
the air out, and encourages

DESPERATION . . . which means "without hope."

A bit way out, perhaps, but the mental picture is worth a thousand orientation talks!

Yogis develop an abnormal oxygen capacity to achieve a state of well-being. Athletes are given a quick boost of pure oxygen to revitalize and energize them in seconds. So we can see how the oxygen supply affects the physical body, the emotions, and the mind—The Three Dimensions of Aerobic Exercise.

With this new picture or inner self-image, one can place the rewards of participating in exercises which promise a richer and more complete oxygen supply into a most impressive perspective:

- More vital physical health

- More positive emotional state

- More acute mental powers

A fair set of objectives, wouldn't you say? But then there

is that small detail of having to take up a very brisk exercise schedule, and there are those, like the engineer, who decide they would rather let well enough alone. They aren't in top physical condition, but they aren't exactly ailing either. The trouble is that you cannot get off that easy. There is no such thing as a physical *status quo* for the physically inactive, as I explained to my engineer dropout. The person who keeps himself inactive, or insufficiently active, is voluntarily stepping upon a treadmill of *diminishing* physical capacity. To put it somewhat more bluntly to those who continually postpone their intention to get started in a running program: "When you decide that you *are* ready, you will find that your get-up-and-go has got up and gone!"

This works according to what I call the Aerobic Physical Fitness Formula. It's sort of a Part Two of the orientation talk to my running groups. Here's how it works. And so you do not think of this formula as in the same vein as my English literature instructor's colorful phraseology, I want to make clear that this is acknowledged scientific fact which can be found in any authoritative book on physiology or in the *Encyclopaedia Britannica*.

The Vital Balance

REMEMBER that you can't lift a finger, blink an eye, have a thought or emotion, walk a foot, much less run a mile, unless you can take in the oxygen you need to turn the food into energy. What it gets down to is this: the limiting factor in how *much* you can do, the work you can put out—is the amount of oxygen you can take in and use. This is the Aerobic Physical Fitness formula:

$$O I = E L$$
Oxygen Income = Exertion Limit

Incidentally, you can substitute the word "exercise" for "exertion."

Everything working in the body, all the organs and processes, the effort of the muscles, is *automatically* at work 100 percent of the time, keeping these two factors in perfect balance. This is the vital aerobic balance which determines your measure of health and fitness. So exact a balance have medical researchers found it to be that many hospitals, clinics, and physical conditioning institutes use it as a health indicator to pinpoint candidates for heart attacks and other killer diseases. Their next step, in an increasing number of cases, is to prescribe the aerobic exercise (with running always in the lead) to revitalize the bodily organs to raise the EL (Exertion or Exercise Limit). The old attitude of letting well enough alone until catastrophe strikes is being ushered out by the new age of *Preventative* Medicine. You can hardly have helped noticing all of the articles with photographs in magazines lately showing men jogging on treadmills with wires hooked up to measure their responses. This is what it's all about. Tests have proven conclusively that those who do aerobic exercise have both a higher Oxygen Income and Exertion Limit. One follows the other.

Enter Mr. Machine

ALMOST ALWAYS during such orientation talks, a new exercise prospect will put this question to me, in one form or another: "If all the processes you've been talking about go on inside our bodies automatically, how are we supposed to have any influence over them by exercising?"

Buckminster Fuller, scientist, architect, and philosopher, has stated that Man is 99 percent automated, and it is a point of view generally conceded to be true. That is why the muscles controlling the automatic inside-the-body operation of the organs—heart, lungs, liver, kidneys, etc.—are known as *involuntary* muscles. But we *can* exert some control over the remaining 1 percent, and fortunately, this gives us control over our thinking and decision-making powers. This determines the goals we set for ourselves . . . and how we use our *voluntary* muscles—arms, legs, frame muscles—to act upon the world around us. The 1 percent doesn't seem so puny if we consider that of all of the three million or more living species, only Man has been able to control and shape the world to his personal specifications.

So we're back to the muscle power of our bodies that we *can* control. And that means we are back to the oxygen supply to power these muscles—and through these, *all* of the inner muscles and organs that govern even our feeling and thinking. When you decide, with your 1-percent control, to exert an effort to do more—to raise your exercise limit—the automatic 99 percent of your body rushes to accommodate you only if you feed it the oxygen it demands. A lower level of balance or a higher one depends upon you. It works forward or in reverse. When you are inactive or underactive, your diaphragm loses resiliency, your lungs begin to process less air, and it takes a lot more effort. Your heart action weakens as it drives less blood with *more* heart strokes through your veins. There is a lessened blood supply to your muscles, and even the blood volume of your body decreases. It is as if the body is saying— "There's no point in keeping up this extra capacity and extra muscle development if it's not being used. After all, it takes extra energy just to keep it running, and this might as well be saved."

On the other hand, dig your heels in for a sustained program of aerobic running, and your diaphragm and lungs, using a lot less effort, begin consuming a lot more air, with your heart pump growing stronger and delivering more blood supply to improve your muscles. A more vital balance is the result, with greater physical limits and increased oxygen consumption.

Add this little detail to our picture: Visualize the inside of your aerobic or oxygen-burning system as being a mine with a glowing candle. The dim flicker or lively glow of the flame is the indicator of your body's oxygen supply and its capacity to burn foodstuffs into energy. That flame is your vital spark and the measure of how alive you are. The dimming flame is a sign of the body's debilitation, which is what *aging* means. Inactivity brings lowered oxygen consumption, and the machinery of the muscles begins to break down, disassemble to accommodate less activity. The bones begin to lose calcium. The process begins to work on a ten-year-old after a week of hospitalization as it does on an eighty-year-old. It even happens to our powerfully conditioned astronauts if they remain inactive during the several days of orbiting. That is why they have to take sufficient exercise. If they do not, the tests show the same effects, with the calcium loss—even in a matter of days!—that we find in the *aging* person.

It is about time that somebody scrapped the generally accepted idea of what aging, growing old, really means.

The Age Trap

HIS PHYSICIAN sent H. G. over to see me. A man of medium height and build, on the slim side but paunchy around the waist, he was curt and incommunicative. If not hostile, then he was certainly resentful. Presently, the situation became clear. He had gone to his physician half a dozen times with a similar complaint. He wanted something to get rid of "that dragged out feeling." He didn't have much energy, but on the other hand, he had a great desire to get up and do things. He was a printer with a job at the same plant for 18 years. He had been married for 16 and had one child, a teen-age girl going to junior high school. He wanted the doctor to give him some prescription to keep him going so he didn't poop out during the day. "A sign of growing older," he self-diagnosed, admitting as well that he had had virtually no sex life for about two years. This, too, he was willing to take in his stride as a "natural aging" sign. He was miffed that his physician had directed him to, of all people, a physical fitness instructor. The thought of undergoing an exercise program in which running played a central role seemed to him the height of inanity. "A man of my age, nearly fifty, running around the streets. I'd have to be some kind of a nut." I smiled and continued filling out the chart that I call a Physical Activity Profile.

"Do you do any walking?"

"As little as I can get away with. We have a station wagon and a sports car."

"Do you participate in any sports? Swimming, tennis . . ." I started down a list which he interrupted with a wry comment, "I leave that for the youngsters who should be doing it—and the *aging* athletes."

"Do you get out to do any social dancing?"

He began shaking his head with impatience, making no effort to conceal that he thought the visit was a mistake in the first place. I let him have it right between the eyes. I had no alternative. I knew the type. He had undergone the usual long-time brainwashing about which activities are appropriate for a man of thirty, which are right for those in the forty bracket, and so on. He was guilty of aging himself, robbing himself of years of life. And I told him as much. Not only was he lessening his lifespan, but he was cheating himself of the vitality, the measure of aliveness with which he was spending the years

25

he had. I told him about a study current at that time of physical fitness performance tests comparing work levels of young men in their twenties and thirties in sedentary occupations with men in their fifties and sixties, and four in their seventies, who were farmhands, construction workers, and lumberjacks. Their levels of performance were charted, along with heartbeat rates, blood pressure, cholesterol levels, etc. These charts, omitting the identity of the individuals and their ages and occupations, were evaluated by another group of physicians. The idea was for them to try to corelate physical performance and body condition with an estimate of chronological age. The results proved—there was simply no way to do it. The men older chronologically by as much as 20 and 30 years were biologically younger!

"Age," I went on to explain, "is a measure that can be applied from several different viewpoints. To evaluate "real age," one would have to consider chronological age, biological age, emotional and psychological age. If we accept the measure of years from birth to death as the only standard, we surrender individual identity. We allow ourselves, progressively with the passing years, to be slipped into convenient slots—what I call Age Traps—representing activities, attitudes, and general performance levels which are recognized as the "social norm." By applying the Aerobic Physical Fitness Formula, one can see how it is that we diminish our own capacities as we set our sights lower. Our bodily processes automatically step down to handle the lower levels of performance.

Somehow—I think the idea of the Age Traps intrigued him—I managed to cajole H. G. into trying a short phase, eight-week jogging program. I extracted a promise from him before we began that he would go through it from start to finish. I had a 16-week program in mind, but I felt I had better get through the first eight weeks before springing the second phase on him.

I cannot say that it was easy or that I performed any instant miracles. But I did keep him going into a *twelfth* week, when I moved him into a full jogging program. Then, the same remarkable transformation that I have witnessed so many times, in so many people of all ages, began to take place. The first sign was that he required no further prodding from me and that he was exceeding the 20-mile-a-week jogwalk, jogtrot, and running schedules I had prescribed for him. At the end of four months, H. G., a much happier, healthier looking, less introverted man, left the plant he had been working at for 18 years. He decided to take his wife and teen-age daughter on a six-month European bicycle tour! After that, he thought he might look into the possibility of finding a partner and going into business on his own. He now enjoyed dancing, even taking his daughter to a popular discotheque to demonstrate, as he put it, "that the old meat still had a lot of juice." He had been bitten by the running bug, the most infectious of the aerobe species.

The Age Trap can ensnare the unwary in several ways. With H. G., the trigger was psychological. It may be strictly physical, as when a man who advances in his job is "pushed upstairs" from more physical activities to executive desk work. Within several months, he may find himself slowing down without ever realizing why, simply assuming, as H. G. did, that this was the natural result of a man getting on in years.

Many housewives whose children reach their teens may find their activities and the excitement around the house gradually quieting down until boredom and apathy begin to set in. This is the time when these women start to pay too much attention to the crow's-feet or lagging chin muscles. During such periods of depressed spirits and poor gland functioning, these signs are bound to be more pronounced. They often go overboard on cosmetics. Their apprehension of premature aging acts to further depress their spirits and lower their performance levels.

For Mrs. W. S., a thirty-six-year-old divorcée, somewhat plumpish but still showing signs of an earlier attractiveness, the spring that sprung the Age Trap was an emotional one. A colleague of mine asked me to have a talk with her. She quickly lost her composure and became weepy and hand-wringing, bemoaned "the mistake I made that ruined my life," and allowed that "at my age, what am I supposed to be able to do with myself?" I made no attempt to console her or flatter her with the usual reassurances that she was still attractive, appealing, and that sort of thing. Instead, I told her that what she was forecasting for herself was absolutely accurate and that as surely as she was sitting there before me, the remainder of her years would be spent alone in self-pity and regret. I told her that just as surely, the choice was her own. That she could make up her mind to live a fuller, newer, and better life; that she could face each day with positive thoughts and think about bright prospects and act to prepare herself for this happier life by improving her physical condition. This was something that was under her immediate control, and it was directly linked to the realization of the life that she wanted for herself. With proper exercise—to my way of thinking, running—she would improve her health, appearance, and spirits and *automatically* increase her motivation to get out and do things, meet people, enjoy herself. She was dubious about exercise, especially running, but in her state, she was willing to give almost anything a try.

Today, seven years later, Mrs. W. S. *M*. is a far more attractive, younger looking, and energetic person. The wife of a West Coast bank executive, the mother of another child, and the organizer of a women's running club!—about whose activities she continues to keep me informed. (A personal aside to W. S. M.: The last thing you or I might have dreamed on the day the rather dowdy-looking little woman entered my office seven years ago is that you would be used as an object lesson and a wonderful success story for millions of people across the country. Keep on jogging and spread the good word!)

RXercise

AEROBIC RUNNING aided Mr. H. G., the printer who had ensnared himself in an Age Trap. It helped Mrs. W. S. M., whose difficulty had an emotional basis. My English literature instructor went to aerobic running for therapeutic relief from emphysema.

To these few people, I could add a long list of others whose need for exercise ranged from *A* for Avoirdupois, that fancy word for overweight, to *Z* for Zestlessness (for want of a better word).

This means that, in practice, the effectiveness of the exercise system depends upon its ability to fulfill many diverse *individual* needs. For a better indication of what these needs are, it will be helpful to examine many of the ailments and health hazards—physical, emotional, and mental—which plague Man. There are some surprises in store for the reader.

In 1900, the records show that overweight was no problem and that underweight was. That there were fewer food calories to be had, and more work calories were required to get them. It could be said that the *Physical Environment* was "leaner," so the men and women who lived in it were lean as well.

How about the emotional or nervous environment? Things were slower, and there were fewer things to be done, fewer things to be wanted, fewer activities. Automobiles were not much to speak of. There was no air travel. Radio was a toy, and television a dream, and not too many people had telephones. Things depended on the mail, which was longer in the coming, and an occasional party was a big celebration. People weren't jammed together on top of each other, dodging passersby in walking, leaping to avoid cars at street crossings. It was not a "nervous" environment, and so the people in it were not nervous.

As for the *Mental Environment*, it wasn't too bright. Information was added slowly from generation to generation. It wasn't tumbling out of multimillions of books in the smallest towns, blasting from the radio, or carried swiftly by Earlybird from all corners of the earth. Education was still general enough so that one brilliant mind might be able to encompass most fields. There weren't signs, symbols, advertisements, commercials, and instructions at every glance and blink of the eye. The Mental Environment was not crammed so full of facts and decision-making situations, so neither were the men and women back in 1900. There was more of a physical *and* a mental balance. Living did not call for a lot of "mental work." The body was kept awfully busy and hardworking.

The leading diseases were tuberculosis, pneumonia, and diarrhea, in that order. The real problems and illnesses were the result of hunger and infection. In an emotionally relaxed and mentally stable environment, hardworking and lean, you can be certain there wasn't much of a market for books prescribing vigorous physical exercise.

Now see how the times have changed. By 1960, we had an exceedingly *fat Physical Environment*. The whole country was like one great supermarket, with refrigerated shipment of food out of season and delicacies from halfway around the world, a food manufacturing industry so tremendous that, as Stuart Chase remarked, "Everybody has to eat hard just to keep the economy of the country going!" So, in a fat environment, we have fat people, and the overweight condition is identified as the number one national health problem.

The Emotional Environment is a very nervous one, fast-paced and hypertensive—with fast-paced and hypertensive people. The Mental Environment has never been so "smart," with information doubling every ten years, showering us so fast that even the big brainy computers have a hard time keeping up with it.

A *fat, nervous, mentally unstable* environment tends to develop people with ailments to match each of the three classifications—obesity, hypertensive diseases, including heart disease and high blood pressure, and hypertensive damage to the digestive system with ulcers, colitis, and diabetes. Emotions have even been implicated in cancer studies, according to several leading researchers, including the famous Dr. Jonas Salk. As for mental health, this has been called The Age of the Aspirin and Tranquilizer—with the slogan "Tune in and Drop Out" revealing a great deal about what we are up against.

In this atmosphere, exercise, more specifically, aerobic exercise, has an important place and holds out valuable benefits on all three levels, physical, emotional, or mental. As a physical conditioner and for weight control. For the discharge or release of nervous tension and as a mental relaxant. It is in this fuller context that aerobic running should be recognized as a preventative and therapeutic measure. Its implications go far beyond an ability to do push-ups or display a muscular torso. Because of this unfortunate association of exercise with body-building, many conditions which can benefit from aerobic running pass unnoticed. This is a subject we now turn our attention to.

30

Pinpointing Your Exercise Needs

IT IS COMMON KNOWLEDGE that there are personality types who fall generally into one or another of the categories mentioned in the previous section. Experience has taught me to think of them as "exercise types." Certainly, I do not mean to imply by this that one or another symptom definitely tags a person for a specific category. A person may show symptoms from all three categories. What I'm really after is to broaden the base for the prescription of exercise.

As it now stands, the decision of the average person to exercise or not is made on the basis of personal appearance. An important criterion and one not to be belittled, but it certainly is not the *only* one. Appearances in this respect can be quite deceptive. For one quick example, and one commonly encountered, take the man who enjoys bragging—"I've managed to keep the same body weight for 20 years. Haven't gone up more than two pounds since my twenty-fifth birthday!" What he doesn't realize is that because of limited activity, his body *composition* may have become so drastically altered that he's carrying around 20 percent more fat inside him than he should have. All of this may have been healthy muscle tissue when he was younger and taxing his capacities. Such a man may be in poor, even a serious state of health even as he labors under the delusion that he is really an example of fitness.

Then there is the woman who is determined to kill herself with fad diets until she slims down her heavy legs or those loose layers around her waist. She may have half-starved herself to trim off 15, 20, even 30 pounds without removing these "figure spoilers." She's burning away healthy body tissues to no avail, because there is an inherited pattern in the way the body lays down its fatty deposits. Running might just accomplish what she's after, without the health hazard she's imposing upon herself.

For the type of fellow who is living off the fat of the land and limiting his activity to reaching into hors d'oeuvre and pastry trays and cocktail-time elbow-bending, the need for exercise is an open secret. It is not so obvious for some of these quite common types. The reader will likely be able to pinpoint the types and even match them to the ailments to which each of them might conceivably be more prone.

High Pressure Prone

The aggressive, extrovertive type. High-strung and hardly ever letting up. If a male, he might be the type in business who is never satisfied that he can't do better and always frustrated about the deal yet unmade, the hill unclimbed, the job undone. If a female, she may be the community organizer or working hard for the distinction, in addition to her activities as hostess and homemaker—in some instances, managing to have a career as well. The steam keeps on building and is given little opportunity to escape from the kettle. Something is bound to pop.

The Anxious One

Anxiety is the key word here. There's always a certain amount of underlying uncertainty, concern with what *may* go wrong. A job which may be lost despite a long, quiet tenure. A sense of insecurity even with a reasonable nest egg in case of emergency. A nagging concern may even include "the frightening state of the world" or the trepidation that a long-time marital partner might be seeking greener fields. The body of this type is called upon to suffer a continual chipping away at the emotions, and somewhere along the line, it's bound to be one chip too many.

Bored

Boredom is the unhappy state of this one. *He* has the most routinized work and life. *She* can go through her housecleaning and child-tending blindfolded. Evenings of TV Hypnosis follow. There is a lot of sighing (a sign of oxygen depletion). Everything seems flattened out into a drab landscape of leveled emotions and routine experience. The real problem here is that the boredom is accepted as distasteful but not really health-threatening. Yet it is. Current studies in the science of human behavior show the importance of stimulation to prevent deepening apathy.

Unloved and Lonely

To be deprived of and feel the need for affection; to experience the loneliness that comes of the denial of this deeply biological urge. It happens to single women beginning in their late twenties. Bachelors in their mid-forties. It is a familiar syndrome for divorcées and widows. They are dealing with strong chance factors in the way life happens to turn out. But there is a certain type who requires a close personal relationship, friendship, and sociability more than others. When it is not obtainable, the burden of loneliness becomes a drain upon the emotions and the health.

Mr. Mind

This is a type, more confined to the male of the species, who is becoming more frequent than ever these days. He is the mental type or brain-worker whose activities are almost strictly confined to his thinking powers. He is the reason why science fiction writers depict the man of the future as having an enormous, computerized head and a feeble, spindly body. An exaggeration, no doubt, but having some connection with a very real trend.

There are other intermediary types, but these are the more common and sharply defined, and I select them for a very good reason. They are subject to *certain patterns of fatigue*, a phrase which figures very significantly in any book on aerobic exercise. For all of the types described, aerobic running is, in my opinion, not only a helpful measure but a necessary one to interrupt the cycle which is invariably deteriorating to the physical health as well as to the personality. In this, fatigue, the most underestimated and misunderstood health symptom of our time, plays a prominent part.

The Many Faces of Fatigue

THOSE OF US who spend a large part of our lives dealing with the subject of physical exercise and the attempt to persuade others of their great need for it find that fatigue is their hidden enemy. Fatigue, claims of weariness, and exhaustion are the first line of defense of the exercise-resisters. "Exercise! You mean get out there and go *running* of all things?" That's the incredulous response to the recommended fitness regimen. "But what I'm explaining to you is that I'm always *tired*. Doing exercise would really knock me out!" We ran into this earlier with the case of the "pooped printer."

The argument seems perfectly reasonable. The age-old prescription for tiredness is *rest*. Here someone comes along and suggests, no, *insists* that the way to become rested is to get out there and run, run, run! Even when it is pointed out to the resister that his attempts at rest and more rest—added hours of sleep—have not dispelled the fatigue, it is difficult to accept an explanation which apparently flies in the face of common sense. The availability of test evidence which shows that increased resting leads to a state of cumulative fatigue—what is known by physicians as *chronic fatigue*—only seems to deepen the puzzle. However, it is one easily unraveled when we apply the Aerobic Physical Fitness Formula.

The use of rest to dispel fatigue is logical, provided that the tiredness is a result of true physical exhaustion. In the early part of the century, when physical work was the rule rather than the exception, the doctor's prescription of rest for tiredness served a useful purpose. But in a society where an estimated 98 percent of all the physical work is done by machines, true physical exhaustion is certainly the exception. As the late Dr. Norbert Wiener, one of the fathers of The Age of Technology, said: "In all important respects, the man who has nothing but his physical power to sell has nothing to sell which is worth anyone's money to buy."

As the countless articles in magazines tiresomely explain, there are all kinds of fatigue. Physical, emotional, psychological, or mental fatigue. But for the person who experiences fatigue, there is only *one* kind. He is just plain tired! The question is, is he right or wrong about being *really* tired? And if he is right, how can it be that his body would respond both to overwork and to underwork in the same way? Now to apply our formula.

It was shown earlier how Oxygen Income, the body's ability to consume oxygen, established a person's Exercise Limit. OI = EL is everybody's Vital Balance. Of course, the balance for a highly trained and conditioned athlete would be much higher than for that of a person in poor physical condition. Aside from individual differences, the balancing formula is the same. And being in balance only means that the person is breathing in and consuming an amount of fresh oxygen equal to the physical work his body is producing. Under this circumstance, the body remains in what is called a "steady state," and a person does not feel tiredness or fatigue. The other side of the coin, the getting out of balance, which produces the fatigue, is what we wish to examine. Let's flip it over.

Jack Spratt is a sprinter, toeing the mark for a 100-yard dash. As the gun goes off and he crosses the finishing line in just under ten seconds, he falls completely exhausted into his coach's arms. Jack is a highly conditioned athlete and the level of his Vital Balance is very high, but he has pushed himself beyond it. He has not been able to supply himself with enough oxygen to keep up his fantastic exertion, and he ended the race with what the experts call "an oxygen debt," a shortage of oxygen in his system. His body had furiously burned off food for the great burst of energy he needed, but the waste, or smoke, in his body had nowhere to go. Smoke is an accurate term, because the body burns up waste as carbon dioxide gas, and without a fresh supply of oxygen, no more energy can be burned off. It is like shutting the flue in a furnace and having the fire choked by its own smoke.

Fatigue or tiredness, then, is a condition of always owing the body fresh oxygen. In Jack's case, it really isn't much of a problem, because he has really used himself physically and burned off food as energy. All he needs is to rest until he can breathe in enough oxygen to make up for the shortage. It is much the same situation for a heavy laborer, except that his exertion happens over the course of a full day's work. But what of Mr. Frank, the bank executive, who comes home equally pooped at the end of his day—and he has hardly moved a muscle. He plopped himself down in his swivel chair, even had his lunch brought to his desk, went down an elevator to the underground garage, stepped into his car, and drove home. How could he be fatigued?

It's easy enough to understand now. While Jack Spratt went *over his Exertion Limit* and could not supply enough oxygen, Mr. Frank, with practically no physical activity, went *under his Exertion Limit*, so his muscles did not work to supply him with enough oxygen to keep up even a minimum Vital Balance. Both men suffered an oxygen shortage, or oxygen debt.

But active Jack Spratt's was a temporary one. Physicians call this short-term fatigue or short-term tiredness. Mr. Frank's was chronic fatigue. With his inactivity, he was continually supplying his system with less oxygen than it required for a Vital Balance. This is what tiredness is. As for the aerobes, man and his mate, the supply of oxygen is literally "the breath of life." Now one can see how completely in reverse is the prescription of rest for the kind of fatigue, the underexertion kind, debilitating to Mr. Frank. The more he treated his tiredness with rest, the more underexerted he became and the less able to provide his body with the oxygen it demanded. As a banker who knows his debits and credits and the importance of keeping his accounts in balance, he was dreadfully ignorant about the size of his oxygen debt. It continued to grow and grow as he became more and more enfeebled.

His dilemma is of the same sort as all of the other exercise types previously referred to. But where his was triggered by physical forces, many of theirs were emotional and psychological. This, of course, squares with the established medical findings when reference is made to physical fatigue, emotional, psychological, and mental fatigue. A common characteristic of most of these is that they are "tired of the lives they lead" or of some particular condition: tired of loneliness, tired of boredom, tired of unresolved frustration, tired of mentally confining activity. He was hazarding "physical bankruptcy."

It is only reasonable that the individual should find such circumstances depressing. The dictionary definition of the word "depression" neatly sums up the problem: "Low spirits; dejection; sadness." And the next line, "a decrease in force, activity"—a related meaning to depress, force the air out, which is exactly what happens to people in such states. They become deflated, deprived of air, rather than *in*flated, which is associated with optimism and elation. So, with ebbing spirits or a search for a way out, they enter the fatigue cycle with less and less of what they need more and more of—an increased oxygen supply. This aerobic running can provide more effectively than any other activity.

Aerobic and Other Exercises

As a PROFESSIONAL involved for many years in the field of physical therapy and health education, I am pleased at the nationwide upsurge of interest in exercise. It is a pleasure, however, not without qualification. Exercise systems with eccentric names are beginning to turn up as frequently as fad diets. They make claims of miracle methods to build impressively muscled physiques and cure symptoms that haven't appeared yet! Much publicity on the subject, mingling facts with such faddish fancies, has left the general public with the misimpression that *any* exercise is a contribution to health and a heart attack preventative. It simply is not true. As a result, a great deal of effort goes into exercises which, in some instances, cause ill effects. Those quite harmless in themselves are damaging in another way. Failure to gain any benefits from them dissuades people from going on to find exercises which are suitable for their needs.

Having taken my swipe at the fads might leave the reader with the impression that he can always safely turn to the old standards. For example, calisthenics or gymnastics, weight lifting, and such sports activities as tennis and golf. I'll have to duck to escape the brickbats, but I must call a spade a spade. These cannot be classified among what I call the life-giving exercises. They do not insure the prospect of a longer life, protect your heart or work to heal it if it has been damaged by stress and inactivity, or protect you from many other ills. They are useful activities and beneficial in some respects. They should be enjoyed to the fullest. But it is only fair to the only body the exerciser has to know what an exercise can or cannot do for him. As for calisthenics, the original meaning of the word, strength for beauty, informs him that it is not a *health* exercise. Nor is the muscle-maker's favorite, weight lifting. Surprising as it may be to some, even tennis does not qualify. And as for golf, my favorite is famous heart surgeon Dr. Paul Dudley White's classic remark that it is a grand way to ruin a good walk.

If this begins to sound confusing, we can easily straighten it all out by providing the reader with three classes of exercise:

> *Isometric Exercise.* Muscle-opposing without body movement. Those "lying-down or sitting-at-your-desk"

exercises which promise superlative conditioning "without moving a muscle." These are the internal stress exercises. Your muscles are made to act against one another or against some opposing force, like pressing against the wall. These are superficial frame muscle manipulators that can leave you overstressed, trembling, unperspired, and unimproved. For invalids or those otherwise confined so that movements are necessarily limited, they may help somewhat to prevent muscles from becoming atrophied. But for someone who can get up and get around and do better, "for shame!"

Isotonic Exercise. With muscle-tensing body movements, the isotonic exercises encompass a considerable range, from general calisthenics, the muscle-building exercises such as weight lifting, push-ups, and chinning, to agility exercises such as handsprings and tumbling, also a great many pastime activities, the likes of dart throwing, archery, pitching horseshoes, and what have you. Calisthenics are the old standbys of physical training. Weight lifting is the last word for the body-beautiful buffs. These exercises can strengthen your arms and legs, your outer frame muscles. The milder ones, of course, are simply half-hearted gestures in that direction. The isotonics, in short, are muscle trainers. They have their use in a fully rounded physical fitness program, and I approve of them for *special purposes*, as I have outlined in a previous book, *Physical Fitness After 35*. I do prescribe some variations of the isotonics for muscle ligament and joint conditioning as Support Exercises to the running schedules. See "Supplesthenics," page 72. They are fine when carefully selected and integrated with aerobic fitness activities. Tests have shown that highly conditioned athletes using only isotonic exercises have no edge on survival or heartbeat performance over the average person.

All of this can be summed up by saying that neither isometrics nor isotonics are respiratory or cardiovascular conditioners. They do not make the special deep-down demands on the most powerful of all muscles, the human heart. They do not get way inside, under the layers of outer muscle, to tax the inner workings of your oxygen-burning machine. My creative-minded English literature instructor neatly summed it up this way: "No exercise has the stuff unless it makes you huff and puff!" This brings us to the third and final exercise classification.

> *Aerobic Exercise*. The oxygen-gulpers which inflate and animate the entire system—get the candle aglowing by expanding the blood vessels and pumping more oxygen-rich blood to the heart by clearing up cholesterol and other artery-clogging deposits, preventing blood clots, and delaying serious arteriosclerosis affecting heart, brain, and kidneys. These are the "big booster" exercises such as running, rowing, swimming, rope jumping, bicycling.

Before I go any further with the aerobics, a most important detail should be mentioned. These top-level energy-tappers cannot perform if they are applied as short-distance sprints, races, dashes, or in any sort of activity which requires overwhelming exertion limits that are over before the oxygen shortage can be made up. These are strictly bad news. Keep in mind OI = EL, and you will know why. These brief, hyped-up activities blow the top off the body's Vital Balance. They leave the body *without oxygen* and are therefore referred to as *Anaerobic Exercises*. Racing over short distances, whether in competitive swimming, bicycle sprints, sculling, and so on, produces an identical condition. The body isn't given enough time to adjust its Vital Balance, so that the Aerobic Fitness Formula is not given a chance to function. Brief performance, either above or below the body's limits, is undesirable. Pedaling at a snail's pace half a block to the corner newsstand on your son's bike would hardly be aerobically beneficial.

The aerobic exercise, aerobically performed, is our objective. This can be described as gradually stepping up heart action and sustaining it at an even, rhythmic pace, sending a rich and nourishing blood flow to the muscles to raise the exertion level and a steady oxygen income to keep it there. This interior development exercise promotes a stronger, more vital, more *enduring* system. It prepares the individual for intermittently high-stress demands, sudden shocks, and grants him a higher level of performance over a longer period of time *without* taxing his body by dipping into reserves. The aerobically efficient body will outperform its competition in two ways. The first, at a higher level with a keener vitality. The second, with an economy of effort promising a longer lifespan. With this as a standard, the author feels less hesitant about

39

exposing the exercise shortcomings of many of the nation's leading recreational sports and athletic activities, baseball, basketball, tennis, squash, wrestling, fencing, volley ball, Ping-Pong, most track and field events, to name only a few. Though participation in these events may continue for an extended period of time, they are stop-and-start activities. Great oxygen consumption is called for in sudden bursts. The heart action quickens, soars high enough to spurt the muscles into applications of power, but just as suddenly, the action lags and the heart decelerates. These are fine activities for bodies already well conditioned by aerobic exercise. They are not rcommended as primary activities in the planning of a health-oriented physical fitness regimen.

Run for Your Life and Health

I HAVE ALREADY made mention of one of my books based upon the isotonic exercises, and I have written a book promoting one of the aerobic exercises, *Cycling for Fitness*. But if forced to make a choice as to the single, most complete exercise with the highest aerobic rating of all, it would have to be—running. It offers such superior benefits that during my lectures on the subject of aerobic fitness, I write upon the blackboard, "Running—and other aerobic exercises." I place it in a class by itself. It requires no special equipment, no special place or time to engage in the activity. It is possible to run indoors in poor weather or even to run in place, if this is a convenience or a personal preference. It demands no special mastery of technique. It has been said that baby's first steps are running steps, with its uncertain falling forward on one foot and recouping its balance on the other. A perfect picture of running. It is natural to either sex and a highly personalized activity in that the movements, weight distribution, bone structure, innate rhythms are characteristically individual. With all of this, it has a distinct drawback. It is not in the activity itself but in the mind of the exercise prospect. I have already made brief mention of this, but it deserves elaboration. Because of outmoded ideas which still stubbornly persist in the minds of many who *need* to know better, running retains its image as an activity for youngsters, track athletes, and prize-fighters. Even among those I manage to bring into my running groups, some of the underlying fears persist. That they are too old for the activity. That it could be a strain on the heart.

If they are willing to put the subject out of their minds, they still cannot escape the comments of meddling neighbors or well-meaning family members who volunteer opinions of imagined dangers. The result is that literally millions of American citizens living in the world's most hypertensive, automated society, in which running can provide a margin between life and death, refuse to test its benefits. How ironic that the danger they fear the most—the nation's leading death cause, heart attack—should be the very one that running can best insure them against. The Boston physician, Dr. Warren R. Guild, who is a confirmed jogger, speaks of running as "living insurance, an investment that prolongs life in contrast to life insurance with its benefits going to the widow." Dr. Guild prescribes running to his own patients as preventative medicine and under careful supervision as therapeutic treatment. One of his patients in his fifties, who suffered a stroke, is now able to maintain a daily three-to-five mile running schedule. A second patient, with a heart condition serious enough to require *12 nitroglycerin tablets every day*, was able, after a jogging program, to reduce the number of tablets to one per month—from several hundred tablets a month to one. This is far from an isolated instance. Dr. Carlton B. Chapman, past President of the American Heart Association, has been running every day for the past 13 years and has publicly voiced his enthusiasm in support of running as a heart strengthener.

I talked to San Diego State College's Associate Director of Physical Education, Dr. John L. Boyer, who supervises a group of 200 joggers between the ages of thirty-five and sixty-five. Among them are those with medical histories of heart disease, high blood pressure, diabetes, and asthma. Dr. Boyer made a point of informing me that he ran at the head of the group himself and was a confirmed believer in the health benefits of this exercise.

This I have found to be the pattern wherever I have taken my interest in running and wherever I have inquired. The very same authorities performing research which involves running and which is substantiated by data from thousands of individual case histories have themselves become avid runners. Dr. David L. Castell, Director of the Human Performance Laboratory, told me that he ran regularly. "I'm really sold on the benefits of the exercise."

The Heart of the Matter

LET US GO DIRECTLY to the heart of the matter so that we can finally and permanently dispel any lingering doubts.

The human heart is the critical organ of your oxygen-burning machine. You act upon the heart for good or for ill to influence your entire system in each of its three dimensions, physical, emotional, and mental. It is a bundle of muscles not too much larger than your fist, but a lot tougher. And to do its job as the master of your blood supply, feeding vital oxygen and nutrients to every living cell, it dilates and contracts about a thousand times a day and approximately forty million times a year. The only rest that your heart muscles ever get—is in the fraction of a second between beats. An American Medical Association publication draws this impressive parallel: "The work done by your heart is about equal to the work you would perform if you lifted a ten-pound weight three feet off the ground and repeated this task twice every minute for a lifetime."

The normal heart beats from 70 to 72 times a minute. There have been many tests with superbly conditioned athletes to determine if their physical training has given them an edge in lifespan over the average person. Even Olympic Gold Medal winners as a group did *not* show any marked differences in their heart action from the average unconditioned person. But there was an exception—in one single category. When examining the long-distance runners, physicians discovered a dramatic difference. *The long-distance runners had pulse rates astonishingly lower than the average.* Many registered half the normal number of beats. Thirty-five was not exceptional. Some were down as far as 30. Dr. Guild describes with some amusement the bafflement of physicians who have never before examined "truly healthy patients."

Here you have irrefutable evidence of the heart-building benefits of aerobic running. The powerfully conditioned heart of the aerobic runner beats more deeply and strongly, providing much greater volume of oxygen-rich blood to the tissues and the muscles *at the same time that it beats more slowly*. This allows the heart muscle considerably more resting time than that of the inactive person. An article in *Look* Magazine on the medical findings of jogging benefits for the heart reported: "More recently, other surveys have proved that even among those who suffer coronary attacks, the ones who exercise regularly after a period of convalescence have fewer later seizures and live longer than those who are sheltered from physical exertion. Although complete details are not known, exercise appears to work its benefits by slowing down clot formation in the heart's blood vessels and by increasing the flow of blood to an already damaged heart. Over a prolonged period, exercise can also lower the rate of the normal heartbeat and thus reduce the workload of the heart.

"Physical fitness experts calculate that if a person can reduce his resting heartbeat from 70 to 50 beats per minute through an exercise program, his heart will beat 6,000,000 fewer times per year. Over a span of years, he could significantly reduce wear and tear on that vital organ that would pay off in a longer, fuller life for him."

- The aerobic runner's heart is capable of carrying a heavier load and spending far less energy in doing so.

- The aerobic runner's heart can sustain far more taxing exertion limits by producing the necessary oxygen for prolonged periods of time.

- The aerobic runner's heart can recover far more quickly from its labors.

On all accounts, each human heart offers to its possessor who would furnish it with *appropriate* aerobic conditioning exercise a more vital life as well as a longer one. The word appropriate is one which bears closer examination.

The Fallacy of the Gung-Ho Runner

I AM REMINDED of the time when one of my youngsters decided to improve upon my wife's recommended dosage of a certain one-each-day candy-coated vitamin and swallowed almost half a bottle full. He was amazed, for all of his good intentions, at his godawful stomach ache. Hadn't my wife reminded him daily of its wonderful "muscle-making magic" each time she popped one into his mouth? All that Glennie was after was a little quicker action.

Running also has its proper dosage, according to the individual's physical condition and particular needs. For those who approach the activity sensibly, the health benefits and buoyed spirits are wonderful to behold. As one who has repeatedly observed such gains in vitality and brightened disposition, I become embarrassed by my own use of superlatives. I find it doubly distressing when I discover that this exhilarating activity is being misunderstood and abused. Many of the running exercise schedules which have been recently circulated miss the mark in many ways. One of the more popular books of the "don't-be-a-quitter!" school of thought pits the runner up against Spartan schedules with a demonic drive that is bound to act against a continuing interest in the exercise. In my opinion, and that of a specialist with whom I have compared notes, the recommended running schedules are easily 30 percent above sensible Exertion Limits. Dr. Richard Morrison, who conducts the running program for the Space Division of the North American Rockwell Corporation, told me that he considered these schedules more like "50 percent out of line"! He cited instances of many of his runners who have injured themselves following these schedules before giving up in frustration.

The loss in self-esteem of not being able to measure up to gradations of very poor, poor, fair, and so on is an accompaniment of the failure which turns exercise prospects away from running entirely. Such programs, though they may bestir an immediate fanfare, eventually end up with a limited cadre of hard-driving athletic types. Those who *need* the activity the most are left in the lurch. There is no need for the runner to be driven like a demon for him to begin profiting from the aerobic effects. Let us accept the expertise of no less an authority than Dr. Paul Dudley White, a founder of the American Heart Association. He tells us that even a good vigorous walking pace, *if sustained long enough,* can bring in the oxygen to step up the blood flow and relieve the load of the heart. Any running tempo, so long as the activity is continuous, is an infinitely superior form of physical activity. Those schedules which goad the runner to compress the time of his performance so that he may be quickly relieved of his daily exercise quota are misleading.

First, they ignore the cardinal principle of a gradual warm-up, one to which this book strictly ascribes. As Drs. John Boyer and Frederick W. Kasch, respectively Associate Director and Director of the San Diego State College Coronary Jogging Club, emphasize: "A slow warm-up is the key. It permits the blood vessels to expand and deliver more blood to the heart." As a long-time trainer of runners, I can unequivocally state that it does a lot more than that. It is a matter we will deal with in the Preconditioning Phase, page 66.

The gung-ho running schedules are remiss in other ways. They encourage an abnormal gap between uselessly high exertion limits compared to those of regular performance. It is a leap back and forth like that of the professional miler who moves like a sprinter. Remember, it is the long-distance runner, with his moderate and continuous gait, who shows the most wonderful benefits of aerobic training.

The Aerobic Runner's Creed

EVERY PHYSICAL INSTRUCTOR could benefit from the trainer's very practical approach to his fighter. He spends a lot of time instructing him on the niceties of bobbing and weaving, shifting stances, pacing himself to last the rounds. The moment his man is about to enter the ring, he unclutters the fighter's mind by neatly capsulizing all of his instruction: "Okay, kid, all you gotta think about now is to dust 'em off and send 'em into bye-bye land."

I also have a good word for my own runners. It is one which even puts my English instructor to shame. When out there jogging, it keeps in mind all of the desirable goals of aerobic running, in which the gung-ho approach has no place.

E for Endurance

Endurance is the key to aerobic fitness. The dictionary definition is useful, since it plainly defines it as the "ability to withstand distress, *fatigue*." To endure means long-lasting, and for all living creatures, it becomes translatable into the ultimate measure of fitness to survive. Of all exercises, only the aerobics are designed to enlarge the capacity—extend the EL through a more powerful OI. To work to build up endurance means to be able to perform more efficiently—do more, with less strain on the system.

A for Agility

Agility . . . quick and easy movements, deft and active, the quality of using the body and its parts, muscles, limbs, and joints, with a saving from efficiency that endurance demands. The development of these parts through running action and the accompanying Support Exercises is built into the aerobic running schedule.

S for Strength

Strength of the inner aerobic powers, which medical science links up with the immuno-suppressive system and helps the runner improve his defenses against infection and disease.

E for Energy

Energy . . . the intensified life-force which the aerobic runner earns as his deeper oxygen consumption burns off his food stores in the form of vigorous activity and a more vital awareness.

E-A-S-E, a provocative word and a useful reminder, but little more than that unless it can be translated into performance by the *individual* runner. This can only happen if the running exercise becomes deeply integrated into the individual's regular daily activities—not as a thing apart or as a sometime thing, but as an activity responsive to his physical and emotional state, the pattern of his daily routine, and the very personal tempo of his life. That each of us does perform according to a highly individualized tempo is now looked upon by medical science as a biological fact of life. Such tempos are known as biorhythms. The great benefits of running are intimately related to its smooth, continuous, and evenly rhythmic effect upon mind and body. The knowing physician and physical educator makes his subject aware of these rhythms and instructs him in the ways of applying them. They are the cornerstone of the Aerobic Runner's Exercise System and its unique Self-Pacing Method.

The Rhyme and Reason
of Your Body Rhythm

THIS SECTION is a preparatory one for the Self-Pacing Method. There was a time when I kept such details from the exerciser, adopting the more common practice of telling him, "Never mind *why* it works. It does, and that is really all you need to know." I did this because I assumed that the authoritarian technique, in relieving the exerciser of details, allowed him more promptly to get down to the business of running. It does, but with limited efficiency, and it does not keep him running very long.

By contrast, those who are instructed on the subject of the body rhythms and develop an awareness of these individual tempos have a decided advantage. I have tested this by dividing new running groups and instructing one half of them on the subject and keeping it from those in the other half. While the difference does not show up immediately, over the period of two months the results are indisputable. The gains for those learning to respect their distinctly individual body rhythms have been dramatic, even beyond the running activity. But the interest and the insight begins with the running exercise.

There are certain questions which I know by now I will be called upon to answer whenever I orient a new group of runners. For example, when I introduce the subject of the Self-Pacing Method, I get a variation of this one: "How can I be left to pace myself when I don't know the slightest thing about running?" My rather playful response, "Your biological clock will tell you all you need to know," evokes more than a few quizzical looks. As it turns out, I am quite serious. The unique time-trainer feature of Aerobic Fitness is based upon the individual's biological clock. Scientists have discovered that all living creatures have their own biological clocks which establish their body rhythms, and it is in this context that the word biorhythm was first applied. There are not only rhythms natural to the species but to each individual. The human is no less subject to these forces. Man and his mate are attuned to the diurnal or day-and-night cycles of the earth. The female's reproductive cycle is affected by the lunar tides, to use one familiar example. Research studies have shown how jet air travel, which plummets the human across time zones, oddly

PERSONAL PACING

Time	MONDAY Energy Level (Check One)			TUESDAY Energy Level (Check One)			WEDNESDAY Energy Level (Check One)		
	High	Med.	Low	High	Med.	Low	High	Med.	Low
7:00 A.M.									
7:30									
8:00									
8:30									
9:00									
9:30									
10:00									
10:30									
11:00									
11:30									
Noon									
12:30 P.M.									
1:00									
1:30									
2:00									
2:30									
3:00									
3:30									
4:00									
4:30									
5:00									
5:30									
6:00									
6:30									
7:00									
7:30									
8:00									
8:30									
9:00									
9:30									
10:00									
10:30									
11:00									
11:30									
Midnight									

Special Comments: Note particular instances when you're in especially good humor, or feeling confident, or sleepy and depressed.

PROFILE CHART

THURSDAY			FRIDAY			SATURDAY			SUNDAY		
Energy Level (Check One)			*Energy Level* (Check One)			*Energy Level* (Check One)			*Energy Level* (Check One)		
High	Med.	Low	High	Med.	Low	High	Med.	Low	High	Med.	Low

affects his body rhythms and so his hormonal processes, emotional responses, and mental reactions. Dr. Hans Selye, renowned endocrinologist, has written of the pace of each person's system, a personal tempo which represents his most vital balance.

Anyone's personal tempo can be charted to find out which time of day is his most active and vigorous, at which periods vitality is low and fatigue sets in. Sleep patterns, work patterns, eating patterns all are affected by the individual's biorhythms, which have much to do with his habit training. It becomes a simple matter for the beginning runner to take advantage of this when planning his running exercise period. Those who, like the harried executive, arbitrarily selected an awkward early period to run and "get the damned thing over with" are unnecessarily hard taskmasters. The odds are that their running won't continue very long, and while it does, it won't be doing them a bit of good.

True, a few people are so fortunate as to be able to go running when the spirit moves them. Their work, daily chores, and activities are limiting factors. But there *are* sufficient variations in the swing of personal tempo so that a little bit of attention to the matter can solve the problem nicely. At the very least, they can get a lot closer to a solution by avoiding those letdown periods when the effort to go running seems like a tiresome ordeal. Practiced in this way, the association becomes fixed in the exerciser's mind, and the activity *does* become an ordeal. To avoid this, the exerciser can get out and run at various times and note which seems to produce the most enjoyable and effective (they do go together) workout. If that's your preference, be my guest. It will do the job. I would suggest for those who like the idea that they pay attention to the daily routine of their activities during an average week and check off their "highs and lows," both in feelings and energy level.*

This is only one reason for the importance of paying attention to the individual body rhythms. Another has to do with the act of running itself. This is brought home to me anew each time I get a novice running group started with the instruction, "Just begin running and choose your own, most comfortable pace. Never mind paying attention to anyone else's." Within a short time, the runners are scattered all over the landscape, each one jogging along at his own happiest tempo. Running under such circumstances is an exhilarating activity and a most enjoyable one. The Spartan types who nod

*The Personal Pacing Profile Chart on page 50 is a form that my runners have found easy to follow. It's little more than an hour-by-hour note of performance levels with a check-off for high, medium, and low.

their heads and mutter about things being "too easy and not getting enough out of it" would be wise to suspend judgment. To heed the professional advice of Drs. Kasch and Boyer: "It is better to exercise for long periods at a low intensity than to attempt to squeeze in exercise at a high intensity in a short time span."

We are not skirting the issue of *increasing* physical capacity. With the Self-Pacing Method, this happens all the same, and without any mental or physical overstress. The step-up into higher levels is automatically geared to the individual's body rhythms. For this reason, the various running steps of the Time-Trainer Exercise Schedules—Jogwalk, Jogtrot and Run —have no annoying speed standards which you must strive to attain from the very onset. There *is* a standard, but it is built into the system to conform to the runner's personal patterns. So when you Jogwalk, Jogtrot, and Run, *E-A-S-E* becomes far more meaningful than a play on words.

The Running Steps to Aerobic Fitness

THE MOVEMENTS of the body and limbs go through four phases from a walking position to a full-fledged sprint at top speed. For the most comfortable, efficient, and easily controlled running, the reader should put all of these strides to use. Actually, everyone capable of running automatically goes through these phases as he picks up speed from slow to fast, with the sequences looked upon as a single continuous process. It is, but if we were to do a filmstrip of a runner in action, we could pick out the four best representing each of the separate strides. They are:

The Jogwalk (Slow)

You have just shifted gear to step out into that intermediary position between Walk and Jog. It's the slowest running pace which can be managed and still not be called walking. There is somewhat more bend in the knees than when walking, but the legs are very nearly vertical. Still, at a distance it might appear like falling slightly forward in slow motion. The foot strikes rather flatly though with the weight on the *forward part*. This makes a fine "resting run."

The Jogtrot (Slow/Moderate)

The knees are higher, and there is a distinctly rolling gait from heel to toe as the foot meets the ground. The pace and the movement of the limbs are distinctly brisker.

The Run (Moderate/Fast)

The movements are smoothing out, and the legs are more horizontal, and the strides longer, to cover more ground.

The Sprint (Just for the record, but not for use in this fitness program.)

The muscle-tensing, absolute top speed in running movement which the body can manage. The body is more erect, the elbows higher, and the feet achieve maximum distance from the ground with each stride. The tread is far forward on the ball of the foot.

The Self-Pacing Method

I REALLY could have begun this section without previously describing the different running steps. If I were to ask you to begin running at a slow, almost rest pace, you would automatically be doing the Jogwalk. If I asked you to step it up a bit so that your pace was slow/moderate, you would go into the Jogtrot, whether or not I identified it as such. And if I suggested that you accelerate and start running, but not at any breakneck sprint pace (which has no place in our program), you would be running. Remember now, we are not talking about the precise mph speed which you are moving at as you Jogwalk, Jogtrot, or Run. Such standards make little sense when applied on an individual basis. The body build, the skeletal structure and various levels of physical condition, and the body rhythms are but a few things which account for the differences. When people are tested on motor-driven treadmills, these differences are readily observed. Some are jogwalking at 4 mph, while others are walking. One person may be jogtrotting at 6 mph, while another has barely begun to jog. Physiologist David L. Costill, the Human Performance Laboratory's Director, acknowledges the difficulty in trying to pinpoint the transition from one level to another and the speed at which jogging becomes running. Statistical standards for research may be justified, but not so when dealing with the training performance of the individual. There are simply too many human variables which are not taken into account in training schedules which reduce the exerciser to a statistical standard. This is especially so in group training among uninformed instructors who insist on applying uniform goals to the group as a whole. Many of the runners move awkwardly and inefficiently at an unnecessarily high energy expenditure. Then they come to take for granted that the fault lies in themselves and not in the training plan and the instructor.

Dr. Costill tells of the difficulty of the out-of-shape person when he starts to jog. How he often finds it hard to keep even a slow 6-mph pace for a distance of 50 or a 100 yards. Running may well be an impossibility for him, but as he keeps up a jogging schedule for several months, he continues to improve along with his mechanical efficiency and overall physical condition. He steps out with greater assurance and discovers his ability to move at a brisker pace, as well as over much greater distances. The same workout schedules which left him pooped and barely able to drag his carcass home he now takes in his own stride, while barely getting up a sweat.

The Time-Trainer Schedules are designed to take advantage of this natural progression.

- The JOGWALK is a fine warm-up, a heart adapter, and an excellent "recovery run" to permit the exerciser to step down his pace when necessary without interrupting the important continuity of the run.

- The JOGTROT is the brisk pacesetter, the leveling off or "steady state" which brings all of the body's resources into vital balance.

- The RUN is the "optimizer," the extender of the normal capacities to higher levels.

Each of these special-purpose running steps is used to allow the exerciser to engage in this vigorous aerobic activity with *E-A-S-E*. The shifts from Jogwalk to Jogtrot to Run are played back and forth to keep the runner going without overstress. At the same time, his capacities are being raised to improved levels of performance. These are improvements of which the runner is hardly aware. For after several months, his Jogtrot is executed with no more expenditure of energy than it previously cost him to Jogwalk. His Jogtrot is at his former running level.

The aerobic exerciser has not been asked to run so many 220-yard laps, so many 440-yard laps, up against the sweeping second hand. He moves in Time-Trainer tempo at his own pace. He can choose to run almost anywhere that is both convenient and attractive, changing his roads as whim commands, to avoid monotony. He does not have to confine the running activity to a rigid drill regimen. What an awful way to treat an activity that is, in the truest sense, a natural exercise!—deeply rhythmic, relaxing, and spontaneous, with easy swinging movements that offer a release often bordering on the euphoric. The Self-Pacing Method encourages a full enjoyment of this activity, with a commensurate gain in its proven health benefits. With the employment of its various strides, the runner may easily step down or step up his effort to attend to the primary objective, which is to build endurance. Meanwhile, his large frame muscles and legs are being developed, and his lungs and heart as well, to prepare him for the next higher aerobic exercise level. The more vigorous body rhythm is given an opportunity to adjust itself without any rocketing overload.

The reader would be mistaken if he assumed, however, that because of the wonderful relief from rigid training offered, the Aerobic Fitness Program was a loosely conceived one. Its effects have been carefully plotted to produce predictable results. It is more precise, though on a highly personalized basis. The Self-Pacing Method is bulwarked by other such techniques as Time Training and Heart Training, which will be explained in "The Aerobic Running Program" section. These, along with the Harvard Step Test, equip the aerobic runner with several important controls to:

- Choose a suitable training schedule
- Determine his aerobic improvement
- Adjust his training schedule accordingly

PART 2

The Aerobic Running Program

Aerobic Fitness in Action

THE Aerobic Fitness Training Program consists of:

Preconditioning the Aerobic Jogger

- Basic Shape-up Program
- Intermediate Shape-up Program
- Advanced Shape-up Program

The Aerobic Running Programs

- Basic Time-Trainer Schedules,
  Phases I & II
- Intermediate Time-Trainer Schedules,
  Phases I, II, & III
- Advanced Time-Trainer Schedules,
  Phases I & II

All plans and phases may be treated as a unified program of graduated progression from minimum to advanced activity levels. Each is preparatory for the next. However, any plan may be singled out and maintained according to the individual's goals and aerobic fitness needs.

Multiples of the mile have been used as the standard in the development of the running schedules to advance aerobic fitness. Such advancement is designed to come about *without* the runner's attention to distance covered. He is to consider only the time prescribed for his regularly scheduled workouts. Endurance is his goal and Self-Pacing is his guide. His motto: "Run with *E-A-S-E* at your own pace!"

The mileage measurement standards apply *only upon completion of the various phases* as noted within each schedule under the heading: The Milestone Test. Instructions are provided in the schedules at appropriate places.

A complete running workout includes Supplesthenics, the Support Exercises described on pages 72 to 73. These strengthen the muscles and joints and improve the runner's agility, representing two letters of the aerobic runner's credo, *E-A-S-E.*

The Aerobic Runner's
Ten Commandments of Fitness

1. Have a complete medical examination before you engage in this or any other physical fitness program.

2. Take the Harvard Step Test on page 63 to determine your aerobic fitness level.

3. Begin the Preconditioning Shape-up Plan on page 77.

4. Master Heart Training (page 67) and Time Training (page 75).

5. Combine your Aerobic Fitness Training with the Aerobic Fitness Diet (see Part III).

6. Start an Aerobic Running Schedule.

7. Master Self-Pacing with the Jogwalk, Jogtrot, and the Run.

8. Apply Heart-Trainer Test for adjustment of running exercise.

9. Try the Milestone Tests only at the conclusion of each phase, where indicated.

10. Run with *E-A-S-E* at your own pace. Observe the workout time period only. Endurance is your goal.

The *Right* Running Schedule for You:
The Harvard Step Test

RUNNING is a great, even a spectacular exercise. I must have repeated this about a hundred times by now. I do so, again, without hesitation. This does *not* mean that you are to shove yourself away from your desk with effort, stare at the suggestion (or the fact!) of bulging waistline, grab up the first physical fitness book around, and go like the blazes. The results of limited activity and The Sedentary Life have not been a week or month in the making. Whether for the housewife and her thickening ankles, or the secretary with her occupational spread, or that of her executive boss, time has figured importantly in their condition of physical unfitness. Time in an active exercise program, however, can be a benefactor. Dr. Fred Kasch's counsel to his cardiovascular club runners tells it like it is: "Time is in your favor—allow at least one month of training for every year of sedentary living—aim for long-term gains in regular, enjoyable training—increase training intensity gradually."

To this I say, "Amen," because it is a policy I have applied with my own runners for years, and with wonderful results. The entire concept of the Aerobic Runner's Exercise Program has been constructed for step-up training from start to finish. In which phase of the aerobic exercise program you should make *your* start is what we wish to find out. The Harvard Step Test, variations of which are used in hospitals and universities all over the country, is a reliable indicator. Here is what you have to do.

Use any sturdy chair, bench, or stool that is just about 20 inches high. If it measures 17 or 18 inches, it's still workable, but that test is a bit easier, and some slight allowance can be made when you arrive at your score.

- Stand erect before it, and count one—place right foot on bench.

- Count two—bring left foot alongside of right and stand erect on it.

- Count three—lower right foot to floor.
  Count four—lower left foot to floor.

- *Count Instructions*
  Keep the step-up, step-down going in quick
  succession. Use the cadence count—1-2-3-4,
  up-down, up-down, up-down, up-down.

  A count of 120 gives you—30 steps to the
  minute.

  Keep that up as long as you can, right *up
  until the Five Minute Limit.*

- Now sit down and rest for exactly one
  minute. Instantly begin to take your pulse.*
  Count your pulse for 30 seconds.
  Go to the chart to get your score.

Reading the Chart

INSTRUCTIONS: *(1) Find the appropriate line for duration of
effort; (2) then find the appropriate column for the pulse count;
(3) read off the score where the line and column intersect; and (4)
interpret according to the scale given.*

Duration of Effort	Heart Beats from 1 Minute to 1½ Minutes in Recovery										
	40–44	45–49	50–54	55–59	60–64	65–69	70–74	75–79	80–84	85–89	90–over
0 – ½ min.	5	5	5	5	5	5	5	5	5	5	5
½–1 min.	20	15	15	15	15	10	10	10	10	10	10
1 –1½ min.	30	30	25	25	20	20	20	20	15	15	15
1½–2 min.	45	40	40	35	30	30	25	25	25	20	20
2 –2½ min.	60	50	45	45	40	35	35	30	30	30	25
2½–3 min.	70	65	60	55	50	45	40	40	35	35	35
3 –3½ min.	85	75	70	60	55	55	50	45	45	40	40
3½–4 min.	100	85	80	70	65	60	55	55	50	45	45
4 –4½ min.	110	100	90	80	75	70	65	60	55	55	50
4½–5 min.	125	110	100	90	85	75	70	65	60	60	55
5 min.	130	115	105	95	90	80	75	70	65	65	60

Suppose you managed to keep up the Step Test for 3
minutes and 15 seconds. If after the one-minute rest, you found
that your pulse was 57, this means you scored 60 and that you
are at about the average physical fitness level. Glance at the
instructions on the chart, and you will come up with what you

*Pulse-taking: Experiment to find the best way to take your pulse. An
easy way is with the left hand on the left chest wall. Some people choose
the pulse at the artery of the neck. Of course, you can choose the wrist
pulse.

actually did score. The story is, in brief, that the *lower* you score, the more in need you are of Aerobic Physical Training and the more gradual should be your approach in getting it. Now check to see in which phase of the Aerobic Runner's Exercise Program you belong.

Score: Below 55

You will want to go through the complete 15 weeks of the Basic Shape-up Program. See page 77. Don't let that bother you, because you're going to have a lot of company, including those who score in the top levels, for reasons which will be presently explained.

Score: 55 to 75

The Basic Time-Trainer Running Plan Schedules outline what is in store for you. But you too must enter through the doors of the Basic Shape-up Plan, pages 77-84. Except in your case, you can shorten the program by as much as 10 weeks!

Score: 75 to 90

The Intermediate Time-Trainer Running Schedules are yours, but the Intermediate Shape-up Program on pages 85-87 applies to you *before* you get to Running Schedules.

Score: Above 90

Phase III, Advanced Time-Trainer Running Schedules, see Advanced Shape-up, pages 88-89.

On the Importance of Preconditioning

ALL AEROBIC RUNNERS have something to gain under the Preconditioning Shape-up Program. Some shape-up exercises are advisable before running in any of the Time-Trainer Schedules. Each physical activity requires the use of different sets of muscles. Preconditioning exercises can move the runner smoothly into his regular running schedule without the usual aches, strains, and pains. Leave this to the gung-ho legions. This running program is supposed to be enjoyable, a lift to the emotions and disposition, a sharpening of the wits. Do not allow the three-dimensional benefits of aerobic running to slip out of mind. I consider running an important emotional and a mental exercise as well as a purely physical one.

Those who plunge right in "fustest and fastest" and push themselves into punishing training regimens are also the first ones to abandon their seasonal exercise intention. It is just as well that they do, because their musculo-skeletal tissues haven't been able to withstand the overstress of an unaccustomed activity, even if their aerobic condition is up to it. This includes those in the Advanced category. The aerobic and cardiovascular boost is helpful to all. But there are other details essential to the lasting enjoyment, efficiency of performance, and health benefits of aerobic running which are to be mastered during the shape-up stage. Instructions are furnished separately under each of these headings: "Training the Heart Muscle" (page 67) and "Time Training" (page 75).

Training the Heart Muscle

AS THE MOST POWERFUL, durable muscle in your body, the heart muscle can use all the aerobic training that you can manage to give it—provided, of course, that you use the Self-Pacing Method to make your training program a genuinely individual one, shaped to your needs and your gradual progression. Heart Training equips you with a simple technique to:

- Double-check your own judgment of what you consider proper self-pacing.

- Periodically check out your own progress.

- Control the development of your heart and heart function.

Heart Training is easily mastered. Moreover, as I have found with my own runners, it removes all the negative attitudes about the human heart and the tendency to think about its condition and its examination in terms of illness and defect only. Heart Training has given them a sense of control over the condition of this most vital organ. They learn to look upon this powerful pump muscle almost as they do an arm bicep. Engaged in push-ups, they can flex their arm muscle and gauge its progress. They cannot *see* what is going on within the heart, but they can *feel* it.

You took your pulse in the Harvard Step Test to give yourself a picture of your aerobic conditioning. That is really a test after the fact. With Heart Training, you can take a more assertive hand in building up and "training" the heart. Here's how you go about it. You can use any of the pulse-taking techniques already suggested. Begin your count—zero, one, two, etc.

When running or vigorously exercising, stop for a moment and *check your pulse rate for ten seconds*. Multiply this by six. It should be at about 145 beats per minute. With some leeway, this is about the top Exercise Limit (EL) that you want to go. *After resting for two minutes*, your heart rate should return to

110–120 per minute or under. This means that your *recovery rate* from aerobic exercise is what it should be. So you have a green light to continue at the same exercise level, progressing as comfortable self-pacing allows. Then anywhere further up the ladder, you can apply the same Heart Trainer Test. If the beat is still at 145 per minute, you've made a fine adjustment and "forward and ever onward" is still the theme. You will want to check the heart recovery rate as well.

If your *heart rate goes over 150 beats* per minute, that is your signal to move back in your schedule a bit. Give yourself more time to train your heart for a forward step.

If your Heart-Trainer Test produces a heart rate of 132 to 138, you're dragging along a bit below your present capacity, and it's time to step forward in the schedule.

To sum up the Heart-Trainer Test for quick-glance reference:

The Heart-Trainer Test

- During vigorous aerobic exercise,
  stop for a prompt pulse check.

- Count pulse ten seconds and multiply figure
  by six. *This should not exceed 145 beats
  per minute for Exercise Limit.*

- Heart rate recovery after two-minute
  rest—110 to 120 beats per
  minute or below.

- If your Exercise Limit heart rate
  is *more than 150 beats per minute,*
  move back in schedule.

- If your Exercise Limit rates
  from 132 to 138 beats per minute,
  move forward in schedule.

With the combination of Self-Pacing, the Harvard Step Test for the choice of a running schedule, and the Heart-Trainer Test, the aerobic runner is equipped with all that he requires to gauge his own resources and his readiness for aerobic fitness progression. The Heart-Trainer Test, intermittently applied during the shape-up phase, will enable the aerobic runner to go on to more advanced running schedules according to the same distinctly individual measure of his physical capacities.

The Aerobic Runner's Preconditioning Exercise Section

NOTE to *All* Harvard Step Test Scorers:

> The brief attention to details during these Shape-up Programs is intended to give the runner complete mastery over his running performance. This will presently allow him to pursue the activity for sheer pleasure with the happy accompaniment of health benefits.
>
> Once mastered, the self-guidance techniques of this section will become a matter of simple habit. It is the most satisfactory and surest way of making vigorous physical exercise a permanent part of your regular activity pattern, as well as a relaxing and enjoyable one and under knowledgeable control at all times.

Where It All Began

In a way, the entire Aerobic Fitness Program is an outgrowth of the Preconditioning Shape-up sessions. These started as once-weekly, indoor progress sessions during which I discussed individual running problems, gripes, and special interests with runners on every rung of the conditioning ladder.

Among the lot were four trained athletes, seven women, varying in ages from twenty-six to forty-eight, five patients exercising by medical prescription, and two senior citizens, one sixty-seven and the other seventy-three (and one of the hardiest of the lot!). Brief time units of running, according to self-pacing, turned out to be the solution in training a complete group on a highly *individual* basis.

Gradually, by trial and error, other features were added to complete an ideal self-controlled physical fitness program. These features, which are practiced and perfected under the Preconditioning Shape-up heading are:

- The Aerobic Support Exercises, Supplesthenics.
- The Preliminary Running Sets (which started it all).
- The self-applied Heart-Trainer Test.
- Time-Trainer techniques.

70

The Preliminary Running Sets were designed as an indoor program. They may be performed at home as stationary running in the three tempos—slow, slow/moderate, moderate/fast. They may be performed while moving in a gymnasium. If done outdoors, a small, solitary area is preferable—a backyard, a convenient corner in a public park, etc.

Experience has demonstrated that the shape-up workouts promptly establish the exerciser's self-control over his own capacities and insure a lifelong habit of running as a healthful and invigorating pastime. Again, *runners in all* fitness levels have something to gain by making this their starting line even for a brief period. For the healthy exerciser, the Heart-Trainer Test is a reliable self-progress guide.

Bridging the Activity Gap

Running is the most effective of the aerobic exercises because it represents the highest continuous exertion activity. It is at the complete opposite pole of the resting state. It makes high-efficiency demands upon the respiratory and cardiovascular systems, and its vigorous trunk and limb action also strengthens the frame muscles and joints.

To go from the resting state into the running exercise represents the widest activity gap of which the body is capable. It is a cross-over for which the body should be *prepared* in several ways:

1. By releasing muscle and nerve tension.

2. By stimulating blood flow, opening up the arteries and capillaries, and triggering, *gradually* increasing heart rates.

3. By flexing frame muscles, ligaments and joints.

Let us proceed to the exercises which are the "supports" for such a preparation.

The Aerobic Support Exercises:
Supplesthenics

THESE EXERCISES are performed prior to each running workout and on rest days between workouts. Most of them are familiar. Several are standard, and others are adaptations from more formal versions. They are a result of trying out the entire gamut of exercises on my runners. I have found these to be the ones which are performed with the least hesitation, and my runners enjoy them most. This is, I would estimate, about five-sevenths of the battle. My admission to present readers—"Go thou and do likewise!"

Do not make a fetish out of precise form. We wish to avoid the strict calisthenic postures. Relax, unbend. Pick up the inner beat of your biorhythms. Get moving without any great consciousness of whether your arm is too high or your leg too low. After a minute or two, every part of you will be "getting into the act" with easy, swinging coordination. When you do muscle flex exercises as well, pick a tempo and "get with it."

The Aerobic Support Exercises are described here, but you will find them familiar enough to perform them immediately. The names chosen for the exercises instantly identify them when they are called for in each workout.

Suppleness implies flexibility, and *sthenics* is from the Greek work for strength. The strength I refer to here is that of the body frame. These qualities are important to the runner because this activity tends to cause stiffness in the small of the back, in the joints, and in the leg muscles. Supplesthenic exercises build up the runner's resistance against the stiffness of too rapid a running start. They increase joint fluid and thicken joint tissue for the running activity.

Supplesthenics relax tension in the vital nerve areas of neck and shoulders and *relieve stress* prior to the run. They cause measurable changes in the heartbeat. They serve to warm up the exerciser, gradually opening up the blood vessels to the heart to fulfill its increased oxygen demand when running begins.

The Neck Swivel (Nerve Stress Reliever)
From a standing position, arms loosely at sides, al-

low the body to sag and commence swiveling the head on the neck. In alternate series, rotate clockwise and counterclockwise.

The Shoulder Roll (Nerve Stress Reliever)
Another one to siphon off tension. From a standing position and a body sag posture, begin to rotate shoulders in alternating series of forward and backward motions.

The Big Swim (Nerve Stress Reliever)
From a standing position, leaning slightly forward in swimmer stance, swing arms loosely in exaggeratedly large, swimming strokes. Again, loosening the critical tension areas of shoulder and neck.

The Boxer (Warm-up)
An exercise for men only which all males are familiar with—the professional fighter's warm-up, to be performed with the upper torso slightly forward in the fighter's crouch and lots of vigorous arm swinging, leg shuffling, and body shifting. Work up a head of steam.

The Kickette (Warm-up)
The feminine equivalent of The Boxer warm-up, it is an abbreviated version of the dancer's chorusline kick. With arms winging outward, perform a continuous series of alternating knee-high kicks. Lots of spring to the step. Not worth the effort unless performed with *élan!*

Imaginary Rope Jump (Warm-up)
You can use a rope if it is handy or if you choose (though taking one along for a run can be an inconvenience). It really isn't necessary. Adopt the traditional jump-rope position, and start jumping rhythmically, with the arms going through the rope-turning motion.

Push-ups (Muscle Toner)
For the male. Assume the familiar push-up position. Body lateral, arms straight, elbows unbent, and palms flat on the floor at shoulder width. Legs outstretched behind and balanced on forward part of both feet. Body untensed but resisting swayback. Dip down, deeply—inhaling as you go. Exhale on the push-up.

73

Keep arm action fluid and continuous, and perform dips at moderate tempo.

The Half Push-up (Muscle Toner)
The distaff version of The Push-up, differing in the body posture in that the arms are tucked under, against the chest, palms and forearms flush to the floor. Raise the body to elbow height, lifting torso off the ground. Inhale on the dip, and exhale on the push-up. Movements are to be continuous and easy as you go.

Kickback
Lie on back, hands at sides, palms flat on ground. Raise and swing legs upward and slightly backward, bringing the small of the back and "butt" off the ground.

NOTE: The aerobic runner has no need for an actual exercise number count. Time participation for each Supplesthenic unit is the measure, and Time Training is the guide.

Time Training

PUT AWAY YOUR WATCH. You won't be needing it after the Preconditioning Phase. Time Training, really time estimating, is surprisingly easy to master and rather like a game in the learning. What's more, once mastered, it continues to improve itself without any conscious effort.

Many of my runners are often accurate within seconds over periods of 10 to 15 minutes. One woman, a mother of three youngsters ranging in ages from four to eight (and an inveterate runner!), is practically a "running" timepiece. She is able to manage her entire daily routine without a watch or clock. But Running Games That People Play is not our objective in learning to estimate units of time. It contributes to the making of the more-completely-at-*E-A-S-E* runner and one relieved of the onerous burden of counting off yards and feet and referring to sweeping second hands.

Time Training with the Preliminary Running Sets leaves you free to pick up the outdoor running anywhere the scenic view appeals. It helps to put the "fun back into the run." Exercise routines which become boring and repetitious soon become poor exercise and then none at all. Running is a naturally exhilarating activity and should be kept that way. Time Training, because of its success with my running groups, has been one of my proudest innovations. I can hardly lay claim to it, because the time-sense springs from the body's biorhythms. And running—running gracefully and relaxedly, for endurance —restores the healthy body rhythms as no other activity can. Time Training performs a valuable role with its emphasis upon the biorhythms. Here is how to use the Preliminary Running Sets to develop *your* time-sense:

1. Run your sets at the prescribed paces, Jogwalk, Jogtrot, Run, *with* reference to a clock or watch. Get the "feel" of relating the time units to your different running paces.

2. Relax and run rhythmically. Allow your body rhythms to take over. You will soon become conscious of your natural tempos.

   Now, run several sets with the aid of a clock or watch.

3. Arbitrary "time guessing" is *not* what you are after! It will only block the natural time-sense.

4. When you are sufficiently warmed up, start your Time Training. Note the time of the exercise sequence called for. Then without watch or clock, stop when you think the running exercise is over.

5. If your estimates are going badly do not continue to press it. If they are getting close, keep up the Time Training.

6. Practice on smaller time units to start with, and then graduate to longer units.

   Mastering five-minute sequences should be your eventual goal. The various Time-Trainer Running Sets are based on the five-minute time unit.

Preconditioning/Basic Shape-up Plan/A 15-Week Program*

Harvard Step Test Score: Below 55
Harvard Step Test Score: 55 to 75

PHASE I 5 Weeks	10-minute Warm-up + 5-minute Preliminary Running Sets =15-minute Aerobic Workout

PHASE II 5 Weeks	10-minute Warm-up +10-minute Preliminary Running Sets =20-minute Aerobic Workout

PHASE III 5 Weeks	10-minute Warm-up + 5 minute (continuous) Preliminary Running Sets =15-minute Aerobic Workout

Guidelines

FOLLOW SCHEDULE SHEET OF EACH PHASE FOR DAILY WORKOUT PATTERN.

TIME-TRAINER RULES APPLY (pages 75-76).
With practice, Time Trainers do not need a watch for workouts. Train your time-sense to be your guide for each Running Set.

HEART-TRAINER RULES APPLY (pages 67-68).

- Check Pulse for Exercise Limit, 145 beats per minute.
- Check Pulse for Recovery, 110–120.
- Check Pulse for Progress, 150 ease up; 132–138 advance.

*Harvard Test Score: 55 to 75—You can shorten the 15-week program according to HT (Heart Trainer) Progress. DO NOT REDUCE BY MORE THAN 10 WEEKS.

PHASE 1 · SCHEDULE SHEET

Basic Shape-up Plan

WEEK *1*

Warm-up

Support Exercises:
- Neck Swivel
- Shoulder Roll
- Big Swim
- Boxer or Kickette
- Imaginary Rope Jump
- Push-ups or Half Push-ups
- Kickback

1st Workout

JOGWALK *2* minutes
   Walk It Off
JOGTROT *1* minute
   Walk It Off
JOGWALK *2* minutes
   Walk It Off

Warm-up (repeat as above)

2nd & 3rd Workouts

JOGWALK *1* minute
   Walk It Off
JOGTROT *2* minutes
   Walk It Off
JOGWALK *2* minutes
   Walk It Off

Basic Shape-up Workout:
  10-minute Warm-up
+ 5-minute Preliminary
   Running Sets

= 15-minute Total

---

3 Workouts Per Week / Minimum Requirement

Rest Day Between Workouts / 10-Minute Support Exercises

PHASE 1 SCHEDULE SHEET

Basic Shape-up Plan

WEEK 2

Warm-up

Support Exercises:
- Neck Swivel
- Shoulder Roll
- Big Swim
- Boxer or Kickette
- Imaginary Rope Jump
- Push-ups or Half Push-ups
- Kickback

1st Workout

JOGWALK *1* minute
   Walk It Off
JOGTROT *3* minutes
   Walk It Off
JOGWALK *1* minute
   Walk It Off

Warm-up (repeat as above)

2nd & 3rd Workouts

JOGWALK *3* minutes
   Walk It Off
JOGTROT *1* minute
   Walk It Off
RUN *1* minute
   Walk It Off

Basic Shape-up Workout:
   10-minute Warm-up
+ 5-minute Preliminary
     Running Sets

= 15-minute Total

---

3 Workouts Per Week / Minimum Requirement

Rest Day Between Workouts / 10-Minute Support Exercises

PHASE 1 SCHEDULE SHEET

Basic Shape-up Plan

WEEK 3

Warm-up

Support Exercises:
- Neck Swivel
- Shoulder Roll
- Big Swim
- Boxer or Kickette
- Imaginary Rope Jump
- Push-ups or Half Push-ups
- Kickback

1st Workout

JOGWALK 2 minutes
    Walk It Off
JOGTROT 2 minutes
    Walk It Off
RUN 1 minute
    Walk It Off

Warm-up (repeat as above)

2nd & 3rd Workouts

JOGWALK 2 minutes
    Walk It Off
JOGTROT 1 minute
    Walk It Off
RUN 2 minutes
    Walk It Off

Basic Shape-up Workout:
    10-minute Warm-up
+ 5-minute Preliminary
      Running Sets

= 15-minute Total

---

3 Workouts Per Week / Minimum Requirement

Rest Day Between Workouts / 10-Minute Support Exercises

PHASE 1 SCHEDULE SHEET

Basic Shape-up Plan

WEEK 4

Warm-up

Support Exercises:
- Neck Swivel
- Shoulder Roll
- Big Swim
- Boxer or Kickette
- Imaginary Rope Jump
- Push-ups or Half Push-ups
- Kickback

1st Workout

JOGWALK *1* minute
  Walk It Off
JOGTROT *2* minutes
  Walk It Off
RUN *2* minutes
  Walk It Off

Warm-up (repeat as above)

2nd & 3rd Workouts

JOGTROT *2* minutes
  Walk It Off
RUN *1* minute
  Walk It Off
JOGTROT *2* minutes
  Walk It Off

Basic Shape-up Workout:
  10-minute Warm-up
+ 5-minute Preliminary
    Running Sets

= 15-minute Total

---

3 Workouts Per Week / Minimum Requirement

Rest Day Between Workouts / 10-Minute Support Exercises

Basic Shape-up Plan

WEEK 5

Basic Shape-up Workout:
10-minute Warm-up
+ 5-minute Preliminary
    Running Sets

= 15-minute Total

Warm-up

Support Exercises:
- Neck Swivel
- Shoulder Roll
- Big Swim
- Boxer or Kickette
- Imaginary Rope Jump
- Push-ups or Half Push-ups
- Kickback

1st Workout

JOGTROT *2* minutes
    Walk It Off
RUN *2* minutes
    Walk It Off
JOGTROT *1* minute
    Walk It Off

Warm-up (repeat as above)

2nd & 3rd Workouts

JOGWALK *1* minute
    Walk It Off
JOGTROT *1* minute
    Walk It Off
RUN *3* minutes
    Walk It Off

---

3 Workouts Per Week / Minimum Requirement

Rest Day Between Workouts / 10-Minute Support Exercises

PHASE 2 SCHEDULE SHEET

Basic Shape-up Plan

WEEKS 1 through 5

Warm-up

Support Exercises:

- Neck Swivel
- Shoulder Roll
- Big Swim
- Boxer or Kickette
- Imaginary Rope Jump
- Push-ups or Half Push-ups
- Kickback

SAME SCHEDULE as Phase I.
But repeat each 5-minute
Running Workout *2 times*

Basic Shape-up Workout:
  10-minute Warm-up
+ 10-minute Preliminary
    Running Sets

= 20-minute Total

---

3 Workouts Per Week / Minimum Requirement

Rest Day Between Workouts / 10-Minute Support Exercises

PHASE 3 SCHEDULE SHEET

Basic Shape-up Plan

WEEKS *1* through *5*

Warm-up

Support Exercises:

- Neck Swivel
- Shoulder Roll
- Big Swim
- Boxer or Kickette
- Imaginary Rope Jump
- Push-ups or Half Push-ups
- Kickback

SAME SCHEDULE as Phase I.
Except that the 5-minute
Running Workout becomes
ONE CONTINUOUS RUN. No
"Walk-Offs" at the former
minute intervals.

Basic Shape-up Workout:
10-minute Warm-up

+ 5-minute (continuous)
  Preliminary Running Sets

= 15-minute Total

---

3 Workouts Per Week / Minimum Requirement

Rest Day Between Workouts / 10-Minute Support Exercises

Preconditioning/Intermediate Shape-up Plan/A 10-Week Program*

Harvard Step Test Score: 75 to 90

PHASE I 5 Weeks	5-minute Warm-up
	+ 5-minute Preliminary Running Sets
	+ 5-minute Preliminary Running Sets
	= 15-minute Aerobic Workout

PHASE II 5 Weeks	5-minute Warm-up
	+ 10-minute Preliminary Running Sets
	= 15-minute Aerobic Workout

Guidelines

FOLLOW SCHEDULE SHEET OF EACH PHASE FOR DAILY WORKOUT PATTERN.

TIME-TRAINER RULES APPLY (pages 75-76). With practice, Time Trainers do not need a watch for workouts. Train your time-sense to be your guide for each Running Set.

HEART-TRAINER RULES APPLY (pages 67-68).

- Check Pulse for Exercise Limit, 145 beats per minute.
- Check Pulse for Recovery, 110–120.
- Check Pulse for Progress, 150 ease up; 132–138 advance.

* You can shorten the 10-week program according to your HT (Heart Trainer) Progress. DO NOT REDUCE BY MORE THAN 5 WEEKS.

PHASE 1 SCHEDULE SHEET

Intermediate Shape-up Plan

WEEKS 1 through 5

Warm-up

Support Exercises:
- Neck Swivel
- Shoulder Roll
- Big Swim
- Boxer or Kickette
- Imaginary Rope Jump
- Push-ups or Half Push-ups
- Kickback

Intermediate Shape-Up
  Workout:
    5-minute Warm-up
+   5-minute Preliminary
      Running Sets
+   5-minute Preliminary
      Running Sets

= 15-minute Total

SAME SCHEDULE AS Phase I BASIC
SHAPE-UP. *Except* that:

1. Each 5-minute Running
   Workout is performed as a
   CONTINUOUS exercise.

2. It is repeated *twice* during
   the workout. Two continuous
   Running Workouts, 5 minutes
   each—with rest in between.

---

3 Workouts Per Week / Minimum Requirement

Rest Day Between Workouts / 10-Minute Support Exercises

PHASE 2 SCHEDULE SHEET

Intermediate Shape-up Plan

WEEKS *1* through *5*

Warm-up

Support Exercises:

- Neck Swivel
- Shoulder Roll
- Big Swim
- Boxer or Kickette
- Imaginary Rope Jump
- Push-ups or Half Push-ups
- Kickback

SAME SCHEDULE AS Phase I BASIC SHAPE-UP. *Except* that:

Each 5-minute Running Workout is DOUBLED and run CONTINUOUSLY as one 10-minute Running Workout

Intermediate Shape-up
  Workout:
    5-minute Warm-up
+ 10-minute Preliminary
    Running Sets

= 15-minute Total

---

3 Workouts Per Week / Minimum Requirement

Rest Day Between Workouts / 10-Minute Support Exercises

Preconditioning/Advanced Shape-up Plan/A 5-Week Program*

Harvard Step Test Score: Over 90

5 Weeks — 5-minute Warm-up
+ 15-minute (continuous) Preliminary Running Sets
= 20-minute Aerobic Workout

Guidelines

FOLLOW SCHEDULE SHEET OF EACH PHASE FOR DAILY WORKOUT PATTERN.

TIME-TRAINER RULES APPLY (pages 75-76). With practice, Time Trainers do not need a watch for workouts. Train your time-sense to be your guide for each Running Set.

HEART-TRAINER RULES APPLY (pages 67-68).

- Check Pulse for Exercise Limit, 145 beats per minute.
- Check Pulse for Recovery, 110–120.
- Check Pulse for Progress, 150 ease up; 132–138 advance.

* You can shorten the 5-week program according to your HT (Heart Trainer) Progress. DO NOT REDUCE IT BY MORE THAN 2 WEEKS.

Advanced Shape-up Plan

WEEKS 1 through 5

Warm-up

Support Exercises:
- Neck Swivel
- Shoulder Roll
- Big Swim
- Boxer or Kickette
- Imaginary Rope Jump
- Push-ups or Half Push-ups
- Kickback

Advanced Shape-up Workout:
   5-minute Warm-up
+ 15-minute Preliminary
      Running Sets
= 20-minute Total

SAME SCHEDULE AS Phase I BASIC
SHAPE-UP. *Except* that:

Each 5-minute Running Workout is TRIPLED and run as one
CONTINUOUS 15-minute aerobic
exercise.

3 Workouts Per Week / Minimum Requirement
Rest Day Between Workouts / 10-Minute Support Exercises

Basic Time-Trainer Running Plans
A 12-Week Program*

Harvard Step Test Score: 55 to 75

PHASE I 6 Weeks	5-minute Warm-up
	+ 5-minute TT Running Set
	+ 5-minute TT Running Set
	= 15-minute Aerobic Workout

PHASE II 6 Weeks	5-minute Warm-up
	+ 10 TT Running Set
	= 15-minute Aerobic Workout

Guidelines

FOLLOW SCHEDULE SHEET OF EACH PHASE FOR DAILY WORKOUT PATTERN.

TIME-TRAINER RULES APPLY (pages 75-76). With practice, Time Trainers do not need a watch for workouts. Train your time-sense to be your guide for each Running Set.

HEART-TRAINER RULES APPLY (pages 67-68).

- Check Pulse for Exercise Limit, 145 beats per minute.
- Check Pulse for Recovery, 110–120.
- Check Pulse for Progress, 150 ease up; 132–138 advance.

* You can shorten the 12-week program according to your HT (Heart Trainer) Progress. DO NOT REDUCE IT BY MORE THAN 4 WEEKS.

PHASE 1 SCHEDULE SHEET

Basic Running Plan

WEEK *1*

Warm-up

Support Exercises:
- Neck Swivel
- Shoulder Roll
- Big Swim
- Boxer or Kickette
- Imaginary Rope Jump
- Push-ups or Half Push-ups
- Kickback

TT Workout:
    5-minute Warm-up
+ 5-minute TT Running Set
+ 5-minute TT Running Set
= 15-minute Total

1st TT Running Set

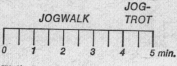

Walk It Off . . .

2nd TT Running Set

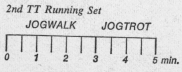

Walk It Off . . .

---

3 Workouts Per Week / Minimum Requirement

Rest Day Between Workouts / 10-Minute Support Exercises

Basic Running Plan

WEEK **2**

Warm-up

Support Exercises:
- Neck Swivel
- Shoulder Roll
- Big Swim
- Boxer or Kickette
- Imaginary Rope Jump
- Push-ups or Half Push-ups
- Kickback

TT Workout:
   5-minute Warm-up
+ 5-minute TT Running Set
+ 5-minute TT Running Set

= 15-minute Total

1st TT Running Set

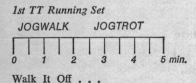

Walk It Off . . .

2nd TT Running Set

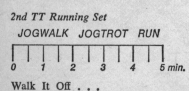

Walk It Off . . .

---

3 Workouts Per Week / Minimum Requirement

Rest Day Between Workouts / 10-Minute Support Exercises

WEEK 3

Warm-up

Support Exercises:
- Neck Swivel
- Shoulder Roll
- Big Swim
- Boxer or Kickette
- Imaginary Rope Jump
- Push-ups or Half Push-ups
- Kickback

TT Workout:

   5-minute Warm-up
+ 5-minute TT Running Set
+ 5-minute TT Running Set

= 15-minute Total

1st TT Running Set

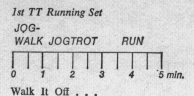

Walk It Off . . .

2nd TT Running Set

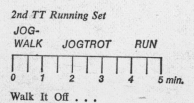

Walk It Off . . .

---

3 Workouts Per Week / Minimum Requirement
Rest Day Between Workouts / 10-Minute Support Exercises

WEEK *4*

Warm-up

Support Exercises:
- Neck Swivel
- Shoulder Roll
- Big Swim
- Boxer or Kickette
- Imaginary Rope Jump
- Push-ups or Half Push-ups
- Kickback

TT Workout:
  5-minute Warm-up
+ 5-minute TT Running Set
+ 5-minute TT Running Set
= 15-minute Total

1st TT Running Set

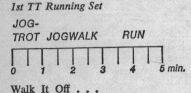

Walk It Off . . .

2nd TT Running Set

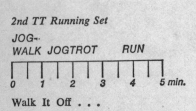

Walk It Off . . .

---

3 Workouts Per Week / Minimum Requirement

Rest Day Between Workouts / 10-Minute Support Exercises

PHASE 1 SCHEDULE SHEET

Basic Running Plan

WEEK 5

Warm-up

Support Exercises:
- Neck Swivel
- Shoulder Roll
- Big Swim
- Boxer or Kickette
- Imaginary Rope Jump
- Push-ups or Half Push-ups
- Kickback

TT Workout:
  5-minute Warm-up
+ 5-minute TT Running Set
+ 5-minute TT Running Set
= 15-minute Total

1st TT Running Set

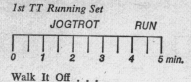

Walk It Off . . .

2nd TT Running Set

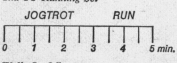

Walk It Off . . .

---

3 Workouts Per Week / Minimum Requirement

Rest Day Between Workouts / 10-Minute Support Exercises

PHASE 1 SCHEDULE SHEET

Basic Running Plan

WEEK 6

Warm-up

Support Exercises:
- Neck Swivel
- Shoulder Roll
- Big Swim
- Boxer or Kickette
- Imaginary Rope Jump
- Push-ups or Half Push-ups
- Kickback

TT Workout:
  5-minute Warm-up
+ 5-minute TT Running Set
+ 5-minute TT Running Set
= 15-minute Total

1st TT Running Set

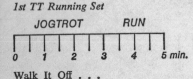

    JOGTROT   RUN

0   1   2   3   4   5 min.

Walk It Off . . .

2nd TT Running Set

    JOGTROT   RUN

0   1   2   3   4   5 min.

Walk It Off . . .

---

3 Workouts Per Week / Minimum Requirement

Rest Day Between Workouts / 10-Minute Support Exercises

PHASE 2 SCHEDULE SHEET

Basic Running Plan

WEEK *1*

TT Workout:
  5-minute Warm-up
+ 10-minute TT Running Set
——————————————
= 15-minute Total

Warm-up

Support Exercises:
- Neck Swivel
- Shoulder Roll
- Big Swim
- Boxer or Kickette
- Imaginary Rope Jump
- Push-ups or Half Push-ups
- Kickback

TT Running Set

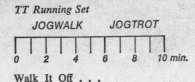

Walk It Off . . .

WEEK *2*

TT Workout: See above

Warm-up: See above

TT Running Set

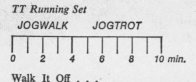

Walk It Off . . .

---

3 Workouts Per Week / Minimum Requirement

Rest Day Between Workouts / 10-Minute Support Exercises

PHASE 2 SCHEDULE SHEET

Basic Running Plan

WEEK 3

Warm-up

Support Exercises:
- Neck Swivel
- Shoulder Roll
- Big Swim
- Boxer or Kickette
- Imaginary Rope Jump
- Push-ups or Half Push-ups
- Kickback

TT Workout:
   5-minute Warm-up
$+$ 10-minute TT Running Set
$=$ 15-minute Total

TT Running Set

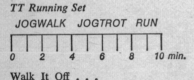

JOGWALK JOGTROT RUN

```
|   |   |   |   |   |   |   |   |   |   |
0       2       4       6       8       10 min.
```

Walk It Off . . .

WEEK 4

TT Workout: See above

Warm-up: See above

TT Running Set

JOG-
WALK   JOGTROT   RUN

```
|   |   |   |   |   |   |   |   |   |   |
0       2       4       6       8       10 min.
```

Walk It Off . . .

---

3 Workouts Per Week / Minimum Requirement

Rest Day Between Workouts / 10-Minute Support Exercises

PHASE 2 SCHEDULE SHEET

Basic Running Plan

WEEK 5

Warm-up

Support Exercises:
- Neck Swivel
- Shoulder Roll
- Big Swim
- Boxer or Kickette
- Imaginary Rope Jump
- Push-ups or Half Push-ups
- Kickback

TT Workout:
    5-minute Warm-up
+ 10-minute TT Running Set
= 15-minute Total

TT Running Set

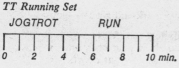

    JOGTROT   RUN

0   2   4   6   8   10 min.

Walk It Off . . .

WEEK 6

TT Workout: See above

Warm-up: See above

TT Running Set

    JOGTROT   RUN

0   2   4   6   8   10 min.

Walk It Off . . .

---

3 Workouts Per Week / Minimum Requirement

Rest Day Between Workouts / 10-Minute Support Exercises

Throughout our workouts, we have emphasized endurance. The running schedules do not appear to take notice of time-distance measurement. The fact of the matter, which I barely touched upon in passing, reveals this as a hidden motive of the Time-Trainer Schedules. It is one which has been built into the running program through the use of the Self-Pacing Method, the object of which is to *advance the runner's capability* at his own pace.

Therefore, the aerobic runner has been running what my inventive English literature instructor speaks of as "the long and quiet race." It is a contest to break away from the former, binding limitations of the poorly conditioned body. The runner who has progressed to this point has been running a most promising footrace, with health and lasting vigor already drawing into view. And if this elusive pair will not be reached by dint of mercurial speed, they will just as surely be run to the ground!

As an indication of your growing capabilities, you might wish to Run the Milestone. Pick any site you know of which measures a mile, or measure one off on your car's odometer as you drive along. Now choose a time when you are able to pursue your pleasure without any rooters to spur you on. You are *still determined to run at your own pace*—but you will find this improving quite a bit. Though Running the Milestone is not to be looked upon as a sign of your success or failure, it is provided to give you another instrument to gauge your progress as you graduate from one level of capability to the next one higher. The Milestone informs you that you are nearing that crossing. Whether to make it just yet is what we wish to know. For this reason, as you ready yourself for . . .

The Milestone

- Choose your own mark and get set—go!

- Sprinting is definitely out. Move rhythmically and allow your body and your time sense to gauge your effort.

- Try to peak at that "steady state" level at which the OI=EL fitness formula works for you. With the oxygen being resupplied, you can go on and on.

- *A mile in under* TEN MINUTES is the limit we are interested in at this point.

Yes, it is simple enough to train yourself to run footraces and to chop minutes off this mark, but remember, this is *not* our goal, and you have not been encouraged to train in this way. If you make the mile-in-ten and your Heart-Trainer rate tells you that all is as it should be, that is what we want. Now, move along to the next TT running schedule. You can still do it with the HT as your guide, and at a slow rate, but it is suggested that if you do not do the mile-in-ten, you remain at the exercise level that you are at for a while.

Continue to run with *E-A-S-E*, and take the Milestone again after some weeks go by. You will pleasantly surprise yourself.

Intermediate Time-Trainer Running Plans/An 18-Week Program*

Harvard Step Test Score: 75 to 90

PHASE I 6 Weeks	5-minute Warm-up + 10-minute TT Running Set + 10-minute TT Running Set = 25-minute Aerobic Workout

PHASE II 6 Weeks	5-minute Warm-up + 20-minute TT Running Set = 25-minute Aerobic Workout

PHASE III 6 Weeks	5-minute Warm-up + 30-minute TT Running Set = 35-minute Aerobic Workout

Guidelines

FOLLOW SCHEDULE SHEET OF EACH PHASE FOR DAILY WORKOUT PATTERN.

TIME-TRAINER RULES APPLY (pages 75-76). With practice, Time Trainers do not need a watch for workouts. Train your time-sense to be your guide for each Running Set.

HEART-TRAINER RULES APPLY (pages 67-68).

- Check Pulse for Exercise Limit, 145 beats per minute.
- Check Pulse for Recovery, 110–120.
- Check Pulse for Progress, 150, ease up; 132–138 advance.

* You can shorten the 18-week program according to your HT (Heart Trainer) Progress. DO NOT REDUCE IT BY MORE THAN 6 WEEKS.

Intermediate Running Plan

WEEK 1

Warm-up

Support Exercises:
- Neck Swivel
- Shoulder Roll
- Big Swim
- Boxer or Kickette
- Imaginary Rope Jump
- Push-ups or Half Push-ups
- Kickback

TT Workout:
   5-minute Warm-up
+ 10-minute TT Running Set
+ 10-minute TT Running Set
= 25-minute Total

1st TT Running Set

JOGTROT JOGWALK RUN

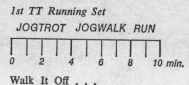

0   2   4   6   8   10 min.

Walk It Off . . .

2nd TT Running Set

          JOG-
JOGTROT WALK   RUN

0   2   4   6   8   10 min.

Walk It Off . . .

---

3 Workouts Per Week / Minimum Requirement
Rest Day Between Workouts / 10-Minute Support Exercises

Intermediate Running Plan

WEEK 2

Warm-up

Support Exercises:
- Neck Swivel
- Shoulder Roll
- Big Swim
- Boxer or Kickette
- Imaginary Rope Jump
- Push-ups or Half Push-ups
- Kickback

TT Workout:
  5-minute Warm-up
+ 10-minute TT Running Set
+ 10-minute TT Running Set
= 25-minute Total

1st TT Running Set

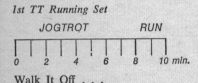

Walk It Off . . .

2nd TT Running Set

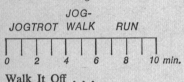

Walk It Off . . .

---

3 Workouts Per Week / Minimum Requirement

Rest Day Between Workouts / 10-Minute Support Exercises

PHASE 1 SCHEDULE SHEET

Intermediate Running Plan

WEEK 3

Warm-up

Support Exercises:

- Neck Swivel
- Shoulder Roll
- Big Swim
- Boxer or Kickette
- Imaginary Rope Jump
- Push-ups or Half Push-ups
- Kickback

TT Workout:
  5-minute Warm-up
+ 10-minute TT Running Set
+ 10-minute TT Running Set
= 25-minute Total

1st TT Running Set

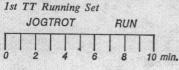

Walk It Off . . .

2nd TT Running Set

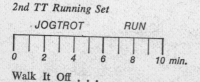

Walk It Off . . .

---

3 Workouts Per Week / Minimum Requirement

Rest Day Between Workouts / 10-Minute Support Exercises

WEEK 4

Warm-up

Support Exercises:
- Neck Swivel
- Shoulder Roll
- Big Swim
- Boxer or Kickette
- Imaginary Rope Jump
- Push-ups or Half Push-ups
- Kickback

TT Workout:
 5-minute Warm-up
+ 10-minute TT Running Set
+ 10-minute TT Running Set
= 25-minute Total

1st TT Running Set

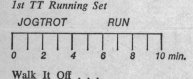

JOGTROT RUN

| | | | | | | | |
0 2 4 6 8 10 min.

Walk It Off . . .

2nd TT Running Set

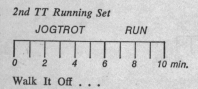

JOGTROT RUN

| | | | | | | | |
0 2 4 6 8 10 min.

Walk It Off . . .

---

3 Workouts Per Week / Minimum Requirement
Rest Day Between Workouts / 10-Minute Support Exercises

Intermediate Running Plan

WEEK 5

Warm-up

Support Exercises:
- Neck Swivel
- Shoulder Roll
- Big Swim
- Boxer or Kickette
- Imaginary Rope Jump
- Push-ups or Half Push-ups
- Kickback

TT Workout:
    5-minute Warm-up
+ 10-minute TT Running Set
+ 10-minute TT Running Set
──────────────────────
= 25-minute Total

1st TT Running Set

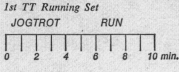

Walk It Off . . .

2nd TT Running Set

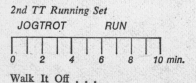

Walk It Off . . .

---

3 Workouts Per Week / Minimum Requirement

Rest Day Between Workouts / 10-Minute Support Exercises

WEEK 6

TT Workout:
  5-minute Warm-up
+ 10-minute TT Running Set
+ 10-minute TT Running Set
_____
= 25-minute Total

Warm-up

Support Exercises:
- Neck Swivel
- Shoulder Roll
- Big Swim
- Boxer or Kickette
- Imaginary Rope Jump
- Push-ups or Half Push-ups
- Kickback

1st TT Running Set

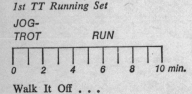

JOG-
TROT   RUN

0   2   4   6   8   10 min.

Walk It Off . . .

2nd TT Running Set

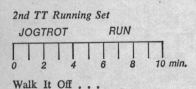

JOGTROT   RUN

0   2   4   6   8   10 min.

Walk It Off . . .

---

3 Workouts Per Week / Minimum Requirement
Rest Day Between Workouts / 10-Minute Support Exercises

PHASE 2 SCHEDULE SHEET

Intermediate Running Plan

WEEK 1

Warm-up

Support Exercises:

- Neck Swivel
- Shoulder Roll
- Big Swim
- Boxer or Kickette
- Imaginary Rope Jump
- Push-ups or Half Push-ups
- Kickback

TT Workout:
  5-minute Warm-up
+ 20-minute TT Running Set
= 25-minute Total

TT Running Set

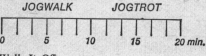

JOGWALK   JOGTROT

0   5   10   15   20 min.

Walk It Off . . .

WEEK 2

TT Workout: See above

Warm-up: See above

TT Running Set

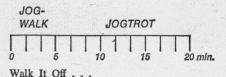

JOG-
WALK   JOGTROT

0   5   10   15   20 min.

Walk It Off . . .

---

3 Workouts Per Week / Minimum Requirement

Rest Day Between Workouts / 10-Minute Support Exercises

WEEK 3

Warm-up

TT Workout:
5-minute Warm-up
+ 20-minute TT Running Set
= 25-minute Total

Support Exercises:
- Neck Swivel
- Shoulder Roll
- Big Swim
- Boxer or Kickette
- Imaginary Rope Jump
- Push-ups or Half Push-ups
- Kickback

TT Running Set

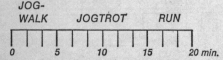

Walk It Off . . .

WEEK 4

TT Workout: See above

Warm-up: See above

TT Running Set

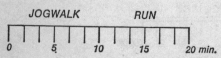

Walk It Off . . .

---

3 Workouts Per Week / Minimum Requirement
Rest Day Between Workouts / 10-Minute Support Exercises

WEEK 5

Warm-up

Support Exercises:
- Neck Swivel
- Shoulder Roll
- Big Swim
- Boxer or Kickette
- Imaginary Rope Jump
- Push-ups or Half Push-ups
- Kickback

TT Workout:
　　5-minute Warm-up
+ 20-minute TT Running Set
= 25-minute Total

TT Running Set

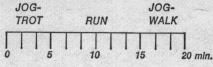

Walk It Off . . .

WEEK 6

TT Workout: See above

Warm-up: See above

TT Running Set

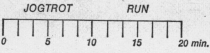

Walk It Off . . .

---

3 Workouts Per Week / Minimum Requirement

Rest Day Between Workouts / 10-Minute Support Exercises

You are ready for another go at the Milestone. This is the distance to measure off and the goal to consider—

2 miles in 20 minutes

"But I did a mile-in-ten. Am I supposed to keep up the same pace for double that distance?" Chances are that you won't have to have much say in the matter. The powers of self-progression have likely raised your Vital Balance sufficiently to move you steadily at this rate, restoring your oxygen supply as you require it.

If your time shows that you have not peaked sufficiently to do the two-in-twenty, *continue on with your* present TT running schedules. Trust your Self-Pacing to bring you forward *within the fitness formula.* Remember to use the Heart-Trainer technique for a sure guide of your physical readiness for step-up efforts.

PHASE 3 SCHEDULE SHEET

Intermediate Running Plan

WEEK 1

Warm-up

Support Exercises:
- Neck Swivel
- Shoulder Roll
- Big Swim
- Boxer or Kickette
- Imaginary Rope Jump
- Push-ups or Half Push-ups
- Kickback

TT Workout:
  5-minute Warm-up
+ 30-minute TT Running Set
= 35-minute Total

TT Running Set

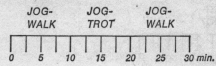

Walk It Off . . .

WEEK 2

TT Workout: See above

Warm-up: See above

TT Running Set

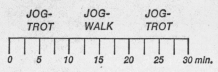

Walk It Off . . .

---

3 Workouts Per Week / Minimum Requirement

Rest Day Between Workouts / 10-Minute Support Exercises

PHASE 3 SCHEDULE SHEET

Intermediate Running Plan

WEEK *3*

Warm-up

Support Exercises:
- Neck Swivel
- Shoulder Roll
- Big Swim
- Boxer or Kickette
- Imaginary Rope Jump
- Push-ups or Half Push-ups
- Kickback

TT Workout:
    5-minute Warm-up
  + 30-minute TT Running Set
  ─────────────────────────
  = 35-minute Total

TT Running Set

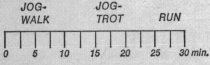

JOG-WALK   JOG-TROT   RUN

0   5   10   15   20   25   30 min.

Walk It Off . . .

WEEK *4*

TT Workout: See above

Warm-up: See above

TT Running Set

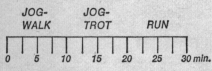

JOG-WALK   JOG-TROT   RUN

0   5   10   15   20   25   30 min.

Walk It Off . . .

---

3 Workouts Per Week / Minimum Requirement
Rest Day Between Workouts / 10-Minute Support Exercises

WEEK 5

Warm-up

Support Exercises:
- Neck Swivel
- Shoulder Roll
- Big Swim
- Boxer or Kickette
- Imaginary Rope Jump
- Push-ups or Half Push-ups
- Kickback

TT Workout:
      5-minute Warm-up
 + 30-minute TT Running Set
 ── ──────────────────────
 = 35-minute Total

TT Running Set

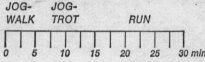

JOG-WALK   JOG-TROT   RUN

0   5   10   15   20   25   30 min.

Walk It Off . . .

WEEK 6

TT Workout: See above

Warm-up: See above

TT Running Set

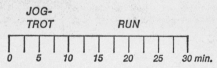

JOG-TROT   RUN

0   5   10   15   20   25   30 min.

Walk It Off . . .

---

3 Workouts Per Week / Minimum Requirement
Rest Day Between Workouts / 10-Minute Support Exercises

Run the Milestone

It's that old Milestone time again. This time the goal is—

3 miles in 30 minutes

By now, you have probably learned enough about the effectiveness of the Self-Pacing Method in tapping your unused, inner resources. At this point in their progress, my runners set about the Milestone with a sense of quiet satisfaction. Another bridge to be crossed, with the crossing a certain enough prospect—so long as impatience and stress do not intervene to press the runner above his fitness formula.

Stay within your OI=EL, and you are sure to do well!

Check yourself out with the Heart Trainer, and decide if and when to go forward at this time.

Advanced Time-Trainer Running Plans/A 12-Week Program

Harvard Step Test Score: Over 90

PHASE I 6 Weeks	5-minute Warm-up + 30-minute TT Running Set + 20-minute TT Running Set
	= 55-minute Aerobic Workout

PHASE II 6 Weeks	5-minute Warm-up + 50-minute TT Running Set
	= 55-minute Aerobic Workout

Guidelines

FOLLOW SCHEDULE SHEET OF EACH PHASE FOR DAILY WORKOUT PATTERN.

TIME-TRAINER RULES APPLY (pages 75-76). With practice, Time Trainers do not need a watch for workouts. Train your time-sense to be your guide for each Running Set.

HEART-TRAINER RULES APPLY (pages 67-68).

- Check Pulse for Exercise Limit, 145 beats per minute.
- Check Pulse for Recovery, 110–120.
- Check Pulse for Progress, 150 ease up; 132–138 advance.

Advanced Running Plan

WEEKS *1* & *2*

Warm-up

Support Exercises:
- Neck Swivel
- Shoulder Roll
- Big Swim
- Boxer or Kickette
- Imaginary Rope Jump
- Push-ups or Half Push-ups
- Kickback

TT Workout:
   5-minute Warm-up
+ 30-minute TT Running Set
+ 20-minute TT Running Set
= 55-minute Total

1st TT Running Set

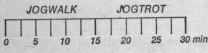

Walk It Off . . .

2nd TT Running Set

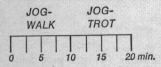

Walk It Off . . .

---

3 Workouts Per Week / Minimum Requirement

Rest Day Between Workouts / 10-Minute Support Exercises

PHASE 1 SCHEDULE SHEET

Advanced Running Plan

WEEKS *3* & *4*

Warm-up

Support Exercises:
- Neck Swivel
- Shoulder Roll
- Big Swim
- Boxer or Kickette
- Imaginary Rope Jump
- Push-ups or Half Push-ups
- Kickback

TT Workout:
    5-minute Warm-up
+ 30-minute TT Running Set
+ 20-minute TT Running Set
= 55-minute Total

1st TT Running Set

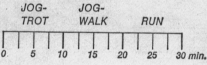

JOG-TROT   JOG-WALK   RUN

0   5   10   15   20   25   30 min.

Walk It Off . . .

2nd TT Running Set

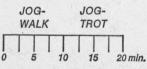

JOG-WALK   JOG-TROT

0   5   10   15   20 min.

Walk It Off . . .

---

3 Workouts Per Week / Minimum Requirement
Rest Day Between Workouts / 10-Minute Support Exercises

Advanced Running Plan

WEEKS 5 & 6

Warm-up

Support Exercises:

- Neck Swivel
- Shoulder Roll
- Big Swim
- Boxer or Kickette
- Imaginary Rope Jump
- Push-ups or Half Push-ups
- Kickback

TT Workout:

    5-minute Warm-up
  + 30-minute TT Running Set
  + 20-minute TT Running Set
  = 55-minute Total

1st TT Running Set

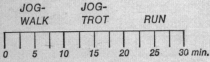

Walk It Off . . .

2nd TT Running Set

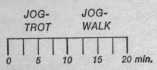

Walk It Off . . .

---

3 Workouts Per Week / Minimum Requirement

Rest Day Between Workouts / 10-Minute Support Exercises

PHASE 2 SCHEDULE SHEET

Advanced Running Plan

WEEKS 7 & 8

Warm-up

Support Exercises:
- Neck Swivel
- Shoulder Roll
- Big Swim
- Boxer or Kickette
- Imaginary Rope Jump
- Push-ups or Half Push-ups
- Kickback

TT Workout:
    5-minute Warm-up
$+$ 50-minute TT Running Set
$=$ 55-minute Total

TT Running Set

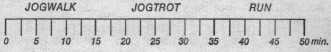

| JOGWALK | JOGTROT | RUN |

```
0    5   10   15   20   25   30   35   40   45   50 min.
```

Walk It Off . . .

WEEKS 9 & 10

TT Workout: See above

Warm-up: See above

TT Running Set

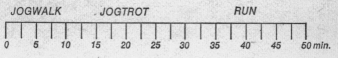

| JOGWALK | JOGTROT | RUN |

```
0    5   10   15   20   25   30   35   40   45   50 min.
```

Walk It Off . . .

---

3 Workouts Per Week / Minimum Requirement

Rest Day Between Workouts / 10-Minute Support Exercises

Advanced Running Plan

WEEKS *11* & *12*

Warm-up

Support Exercises:

- Neck Swivel
- Shoulder Roll
- Big Swim
- Boxer or Kickette
- Imaginary Rope Jump
- Push-ups or Half Push-ups
- Kickback

TT Workout:
  5-minute Warm-up
+ 50-minute TT Running Set
= 55-minute Total

TT Running Set

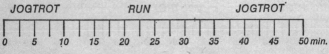

JOGTROT   RUN   JOGTROT

| | | | | | | | | | | | | | | | | | | | |
0   5   10   15   20   25   30   35   40   45   50 min.

Walk It Off . . .

---

3 Workouts Per Week / Minimum Requirement

Rest Day Between Workouts / 10-Minute Support Exercises

Clothing and Climate

THE RULES ARE SIMPLE and few under this heading, at least in the way I deal with the subjects. Reasonableness, comfort, and good sense are what is called for. Pay no mind to those who insist that you require "special running shoes" and "special running clothes," that you should "oil your skin". Nonsense. As for clothing, this is all you need:

> Wear comfortable, well-fitting shoes with rubber soles. They should have good arch support but have maximum flexibility. Sneakers are fine, but for running continuously, I would recommend the heavier, sturdier soled type and not the tennis sneaker. Be certain that the laces are securely tied and that they are not too constricting. Well-fitting, incidentally, means with an allowance for an extra pair of white socks. I do not recommend the bulky kind because the underfoot sometimes rubs back and forth against the sock when perspired.

> Apply talc liberally wherever you know sweating may be a problem. Men have more difficulty in this because they sweat more profusely. Constitutionally, a woman does not perspire as much as a man, and she should make allowances for this by wearing generally lighter clothes to assist in the heat-escape from her body as she runs.

> Clothing, tops and bottoms, should be loose fitting for both sexes, so as not to impede circulation, but *not* ill fitting. Avoid jackets with rubberized wristbands and, similarly, sweat pants with such anklebands. Do *not* use "wind breaker" type jackets or other specially treated materials which do not permit body heat to filter through.

"Getting up a good sweat" is too loosely used an expression. Excessive sweating is not necessarily a sign of "a good workout." One may have been overstressing, moving inefficiently; the clothing may not have allowed the body to cool

123

off. The temperature may have been too hot for a run. As a rule, I suggest that my runners cancel their workout if the summer heat rises above 88°. It is wiser and more comfortable to wait for the cool of the evening.

Excessive sweating depletes the body of too much fluid and too much salt. And do *not* heed the "expert" who tells you to swallow salt tablets like peppermint candy. They may give you a stomachache. They affect many people in that way. If you are going to take them, do not take them on an empty stomach, and drink lots of water. Do not drink excessively before or during a workout to avoid a feeling of overfullness. But water should *not* be withheld from those profusely sweating from vigorous activity. Water is absolutely essential, and its absence can do damage to the system. Withholding it is *not* going to take weight off, because these body fluids will be replaced. As an afterthought about the salt tablets, you can make up for the drain of salts in the body by a liberal use of the saltshaker during regular mealtimes.

There is little reason why you cannot run in the coldest weather if the proper precautions are taken. Warm clothing, in layers, preferably. Good warm gloves which are not too tight at the wrists. A hood which joins with the jacket to keep out neck drafts, and a towel, as a muffler, for further security. If there is a bitter wind, a face mask will be needed. Your head and ears should be well covered. A full jacket is preferable to a half or waistband jacket to keep out the chill from the lower back and kidney area.

Two points to remember about running in cold weather. One, you should take your warm-up with the Support Exercises indoors before you dash out into the cold. This warm-up will get you started fast. A warm-up does *not* mean a state of flowing perspiration! Avoid abrupt changes in temperature. And two, upon concluding your run, do not allow yourself to cool off too fast.

As for rain, snow, sleet, or other inclemencies, which fail to stop the "valiant mailman," I say avoid them. Turn to the Preconditioning Phase and do the Support Exercises and Preliminary Running Sets indoors until another and a better day comes along. Bad weather means wet and sleety streets and muddy ground. In running, slips *do* count.

Women in the Running

IT IS THE ENDURANCE which makes the runner the hardiest of all human specimens. Among my running groups over the years, there have been quite a few women, deceptively ultra-feminine, who could run circles around a goodly percentage of the males. They will not go faster over the shorter distances, but over the long haul, they make a wonderful showing—so much so that it is positively embarrassing to many of the strapping males who like to look upon themselves as prototypes of "the stronger sex." Medical science now informs us that the shoe should be on the other (runner's) foot!

Nature is the ultimate decision-maker, and by her definition, it is strength and durability which are the ultimate survival measures, and in these categories, woman takes the lead. I am her enthusiastic rooter because once she takes to something, she stays with it (contrary to popular opinion). Running is one such example. In many ways, it is an ideal activity for her.

Once rid of the restriction of her movements, which I consider more a social imposition rather than a biological disadvantage, her natural grace and fine coordination help her to take to running as easily as the proverbial duck takes to water. Also, on the basis of observation, I would say that her aerobic system is superior to the male's.

The benefits of running of special interest to women are many. The improved circulation does wonders for her complexion and to stave off the unsightly varicose veins. Slimness of figure and shapeliness of leg cannot be preserved or restored by diet alone. Running performs wonders for the figure, and many years ago, when I operated New York's Strength and Health Gymnasiums, I prepared special running exercises for eight Radio City Music Hall Rockettes who came to me for figure conditioning. Running does *not,* as many people believe, tend to develop muscularity in women. The large dancer's calf is a result of the abnormal placement of the full body weight upon the toe and ball-of-foot position. The proper running position employs almost all of the foot except for the extreme heel and end. Women will find running the finest of all leg trimmers—from thigh to calf to ankle.

There was no reason for me to set up special running schedules for women. They may perform any and all of the running schedules as described. The two exceptions appear in the Support Exercises. The Boxer is one, and I confine it to the male of the species because of its unfeminine movements. I do not recommend the conventional Push-up exercise but have included The Half Push-up for women. It is a fine bust shaper.

Note should be made of the difference in heartbeat rate for women. It is slightly higher than for men, but the Heart-Trainer Test will still serve as an adequate indicator.

Running from Illness

MUCH IS presently being reported about the wonderful, some even use the word "magical," properties of running as a cure-all: case histories of the "running" recoveries of a Mr. R. B. from lung collapse, a Miss F. L. from asthma, Mrs. C. M. from colitis. Volumes could be filled with such case histories, the listed ailments reading like a medical dictionary of "all the ills the flesh is heir to"— coronary heart disease, high blood pressure or hypertension, diabetes, skin allergies, anemia, emphysema, neuritis and neuralgia, ulcers, migraines, nervous tics—and the results being either recoveries or decided improvement and relief from symptoms.

In a way, I find the publication of information of this kind saddening. It is an indication that the *real* message which needs to be communicated to multimillions of Americans on the borderline of health is being missed. One would have hoped that the pervasive cure-all approach to medical health had gone out with the bottled elixirs.

To treat running as if it were something inside a bottle or tablet (or between the covers of a book) exposes it to faddism, which totters upon the whims of public fancy until the next bright idea comes along. If this were to happen to running as an exercise, it would indeed be a tragic loss for public health and the field of *preventative* medicine. How ironic that it needs to be pointed out that running is not in a bottle or tablet, but inside Man, inside his limbs since the dawn of creation. *That the miracle properties are those inherent in his own body* if he would but put them to work to reach and to use the deepest of his capacities. That illness and debilitation follow inactivity, the sedentary, stressful life. That this is a pernicious cycle which, once taken up, perpetuates itself. The benefits of running, cited in cases of relief and cure, demonstrate beyond all dispute that the powers of restoration and reinvigoration are in ourselves. "Physician, cure thyself." Hippocrates indeed knew whereof he spoke.

Nothing could be as important as a renewal of this fundamental verity in our high-pressure, overly mechanized age with its dependence upon therapeutic rather than preventative medicine. These case histories suggest a "running" away from illness, important, even critical, to the individuals so afflicted. But illness, incapacity, are after-the-fact conditions—after the damage has been done. *Running toward health* as a positive and preventative measure is the attitude which must be instilled if we are to escape the crippling national pandemic caused by the limited use or disuse of the body's full capacities.

It is for this reason that I prefer to look upon the various diseases and infirmities not as separate entities but as part of an overall three-dimensional pattern in which relation aerobic running can perform a valuable *guardian function*.

Run for Your Circulation
When you run, you are acting upon the critical organs of the cardiovascular system, and you are guarding yourself against diseases of the heart, the veins, and arteries, cerebral hemorrhage, and many of the circulatory ills including high blood pressure or hypertension.

Run for Your Respiration
When you run, you are building up your respiratory system and acting against the lung diseases and such impairments as emphysema, bronchitis, asthma.

Run for Your Digestion
When you run, you are defending yourself against the common ailments related to the digestive system: ulcers, colitis, diabetes, constipation.

Run for Your Motor Action
When you run, you are strengthening your body frame, joints and ligaments, the motor nerves, triggering your muscle movements. You are protecting yourself against the onset of the joint-stiffening diseases, neuritis and neuralgia and backache.

Run for Your Emotions
When you run, you are acting upon the glands and nerves controlling the emotions and the senses which make possible your response to the world around you.

The average person does not wish to go into the details of the symptoms and the physiology of each of the diseases or ailments. If he does, in this or that instance, the details quickly pass out of his mind. But this grouping does *not*, with the result that any ailment mentioned is automatically placed under one of these headings.

Aside from helping to remove the mystery attending so many human ills, it gives the aerobic runner a sense of control over what goes on inside him. He recognizes running not as a fad or a miracle device but as a sound *preventative* as well as a corrective measure in the preservation of his health and his life.

Running as Therapeutic Treatment

IF YOU ARE presently under medical treatment, talk to your personal physician about the possible inclusion of a regular exercise program as part of this treatment.

Under such circumstances, medical supervision is essential. Periodic checkups are in order to help keep apace of the improvement of your condition. A consistent finding in regard to the benefits of aerobic exercise is the need for scaling down medication dosage. This is true among many diabetic, cardiac, and high blood pressure patients, as well as those with less serious ailments.

For the Runner under Medical Treatment

- He must have professional medical supervision.

- He must respect the importance of the slow and gradual warm-up.

- He must exercise in intervals and have the benefit of the Heart Trainer Test to check his exercise limits and recovery rates.

- He must exercise with regularity and emphasize the continuous rhythms of aerobic activity.

The physician may wish to recommend a scaled-down version of the Preconditioning Exercises or retain the present schedule with longer recovery periods between the Preliminary Running Sets. Many patients have progressed from this level of the schedule right on through the Intermediate Time-Trainer Phases. In one instance, that of a retired architect, a cardiac patient in his late sixties, he went on beyond Phase III and a running program of sixty miles per week! His running had sufficiently enlarged the hardening arteries around his heart to provide an increase in blood supply to normal levels.

Many victims of angina pectoris, chest pain resulting from a diminished blood supply to the heart, are benefited by running programs such as those initiated by Drs. Kasch and Boyer.

Those suffering from the joint diseases require special rehabilitative exercises which are not within the province of this book. Many can be greatly benefited by improving overall circulation, but inflamed joints should never be exercised until all swelling and signs of inflammation disappear.

The overweight condition is a special problem because (1) it is considered the number one public health problem, and (2) it has been identified as a complicating and high risk factor in all of the high mortality diseases.

Aerobic running has much to offer the overweight person in conjunction with a sensible dietary regimen. The reader's attention is drawn to "The Aerobic Energy-Control Diet," Part III of this book, for this purpose. A few thoughts on the peculiarities of the overweight condition as it relates to "the underexercised" are apropos here.

The Fat Cycle

THE OVERWEIGHT CONDITION strikes close to home for a large percentage of those in each of my new running groups. I bring up the subject with the statement—"The bi-cycle of physical *un*fitness is made up of the FATigue cycle and the Fat cycle. A turn of one manipulates the other."

Fatigue or tiredness, whatever its cause, reduces physical activity. This means less food burned as energy and more stored within the body. The fat tissues are stored (though a useless deadweight in this form) energy. The same amount of food is eaten, and generally more, because inactivity tends to upset the appetite control. There is such a control mechanism in the brain, and it is supposed to trigger feelings of hunger for food—only in equal proportion to the amount of energy the body has used in running itself (it costs about 75 calories per hour even while you are sleeping) and the bigger expenditures that come from physical activity. Continuous running can burn up more calories than any other physical activity.

In the poorly conditioned, inactive person, appetite seems to develop a mind of its own! And the more it is taunted, tempted, and partially starved with unbalanced diets, the more unruly it becomes—until we are dealing with "the runaway appetite."

So the cycle goes from fatigue and inactivity to more eating and overweight. And to make it all the worse, for those who are overweight and eat less—their inactive bodies turn it into fat more efficiently! There is more to the picture than the consideration of the body as a simple energy machine—food energy in and exercise energy out.

The picture is not too hopeful for the inactive underexercised dieter, but it brightens up considerably for the dieter who decides on aerobic running as well! The Energy-Control Diet returns the reins of the runaway appetite to the hands of the exerciser. What is more, it promises him more than the temporary control of the usual diet-and-bodyweight seesaw.

Other aerobic exercisers will wish to turn to the Energy-Control Diet because it has been developed, with built-in modifications, as a Fitness Diet. You might say that the Energy-Control Diet has *dual* controls. One set RD, Reducing Diet—the other FD, Fitness Diet.

PART 3

The Aerobic Energy-Control Diet

The Candidates
for Diet and Fitness

BY FAR the largest number of people attracted to running or to any physical fitness program are drawn to it because of the accumulation of excess bodyweight. I have classified those among my running groups in this way: 6 percent to 16 percent over their normal bodyweight; 16 percent and over. There is another class whom I do not consider overweight in any but the strictest sense: those who are the normals in the 0 percent to 6 percent overweight category, but whose flabby body tissues identify them as fitness cases. They are in need of the firming up of a physical fitness program. Much of their former muscle tissue has been converted into fat because of inactivity. I do not mean that the Six and Sixteen Plussers are *not* fitness cases. But they require a Reducing Diet (RD) along *with* a fitness program. The Zero Plussers need special attention to what they eat as well, because exercise and diet are two sides of the same coin, but a Fitness Diet (FD) is what they require. Substantial weight loss is not for them. They need a firming up of the fat into solid muscle. The weight record charts on my own runners have taught me to line up the candidates for diet and fitness in this order:

The 0 Plussers   0 percent–6 percent overweight
in need of FD (*Fitness Diet*)

The 6 Plussers   6 percent–16 percent overweight
in need of RD (*Reducing Diet*)

The 16 Plussers   16 percent + overweight
in need of RD+ (*Reducing Diet, more strictly applied*)

Which are you? If you have any doubt, you will have an opportunity to check it out as we go along.

Food Energy
and Exercise Energy

LOSING POUNDS and gaining them back, trying this diet and the other diet. It was the main topic of conversation among my running groups, and it presently became a matter of interest and concern to me. Constant fluctuations of bodyweight are unhealthy. As a matter of fact, medical research has shown that a moderate amount of overweight (ten pounds, perhaps fifteen if the frame is large enough) is less destructive to the system than the punishing weight-change pendulum swinging back and forth and upsetting the body's Vital Balance. Also, the nutritional balance of the body is a delicate one. It may be depleted of any one of some 55 necessary nutrients which the system needs. For this reason, fad diets can be damaging, even dangerous to health.

As a physical trainer, I am aware always that the common coin of exercise—planned physical activity—is *energy*. The aerobic runner seeks to consume more oxygen in order to burn up his food stores and produce this energy. If we are more active, vigorously as in aerobic running, we spend more energy. If we are inactive or barely so, we spend less. Since we continue to eat all the time, three or more meals and goodies a day, we are saving up loads of energy—which our body stores up in the form of fats. So when you see a really obese man or woman, you are looking at great bulging stores of unused energy that excessively pad the system and act as a drag on it.

All of the dieters who talk in pounds and calories are really playing the Energy Game, but they do not think of it in that way. Of course, they know that exercise "burns up calories" (which is only a measure of the amount of energy), but still, diet remains one subject for them and exercise another. For the simple reason, as they will tell you, "You can't really lose weight by doing exercise." And they will immediately offer examples of the number of times a man would have to run up and down the Washington Monument in order to work off the energy in one pat of butter! Or that it would take seven hours of playing tennis to lose a single pound—3,500 calories. And so on. So if you want to lose weight, why exercise? It is easy, by the same token, to point out that a vigorous walk each evening could use up 300 calories of energy and cause a weight loss of a pound per week, or 52 pounds a year! But that would be playing the game their way, and there is a lot more to it.

For one thing, as I began to describe earlier, there is the matter of the appestat. It is an automatic appetite control in the part of the brain called the hypothalamus. Its purpose is to keep in balance the amount of food energy you consume with the amount of energy used up as activity. In a healthy, well-conditioned person, this appestat functions well. As a person becomes inactive and loses his Vital Balance, this mechanism goes off and the fat cycle begins. The amount of food consumed has no relation to what is used, and the fat stores (unused energy) grow and grow. What's more, the system of a person who is much overweight produces fats much more efficiently. In comparing two people, one heavy and one thin, eating the same foods in amount and kind—the heavy one gets much the worst of the deal. And if he loses weight by dieting, he will gain back his weight faster a second time. Will dieting without exercise help him? To make a shameless pun—fat chance!

Diet deals with taking food energy into the body. Exercise deals *not only* with discharging such food energy as activity energy. The exercise raises the level of the body's Vital Balance. This changes the way the body processes the food taken in and also the way it restores the appestat, the appetite control. The healthy and well-conditioned person has *less* of a problem with a desire to eat. As he works or is active, his body craves food to replace exactly the energy he used up. When he is inactive, he feels satisfied with little.

The poorly conditioned, overweight person must gain control of both levers—food energy on the one side and activity energy on the other—if he is to maintain a normal weight *and* a normal appetite. *Energy* must be *controlled* in the form of food intake and exercise output.

The Self-Pacing Method and the Heart Trainer were designed to give the runner control of his exercise energy. A complementary diet was needed to give the runner control of his food energy. These combined would give him Energy Control.

The Energy Food

TO BE TECHNICAL about it, there is only one food which can be properly classified as "the energy food." Sound nutrition demands a diet balanced in proteins, fats, and carbohydrates—but only the *carbohydrates* are referred to in this way by nutritionists. The proteins and fats are used to build and support the body tissues. The fats, which also contribute to the digestive process, may be *converted* into energy. Some of the proteins can as well, but the carbohydrates are the quick-energy food. They are found in the starches, such foods as breads and rolls, cakes, potatoes, noodles, as well as the sugar foods—candy, preserves, syrups, and soft drinks. Carbohydrates must be used as energy, and if they are not—they are converted into fats; and here we have the first clue to the development of The Fat Society.

A push-button nation of tremendous abundance providing an incredibly high-energy diet. Its inactive people storing up the carbohydrate energy as useless depot fats. So many of the carbohydrate foods are eaten not to satisfy hunger but for taste stimulation. One psychologist has referred to them as "consolation or reward foods." They are the treats—cakes, pastries, assorted goodies and desserts at parties and celebrations, coffee klatches, the tempters at restaurant and home meals, and the consolers in moments of boredom, loneliness, and despair. They become an increasing problem as the overweight load grows. Intermittent diets and the attempt to deny the appetite for carbohydrates only deepens the craving for them. Dr. Walter Bloom, Director of Medical Education in Atlanta's Piedmont Hospital, in his remarks before a symposium on the Prevention of Obesity, stated about most obese patients that they are "definitely addicted to the carbohydrate and are excessive carbohydrate eaters." (He calls them "carboholics.")

The problem in handling carbohydrates is not limited to those who have very serious weight problems. Dr. Herta Spencer, Chief of the Metabolic Section at Illinois Veterans Administration Hospital, has referred to studies of people with perfectly normal weight who were able to maintain or lose weight on a diet high in protein, while they gained weight in a diet high in carbohydrates. The effectiveness of a "low-energy diet" developed at Michigan State University was proven both

138

there and at Cornell University. It was high in protein, moderate in fat, and low in the carbohydrates. More than one half of the energy in the diet came from fats, which are slower to digest and give more lasting satisfaction. Seven of the tested subjects lost 19 to 37 pounds at the end of 16 weeks. A similar diet limiting carbohydrates and tested at Cornell University showed that 10 subjects lost between 9 and 23.5 pounds in 8 to 9 weeks. This weight was lost without any looseness of skin, flabbiness of tissue, and without any special desire for food between meals.

Still, where diet alone was used as the measure to control weight, the long-range results were dismal. A definitive study by A. J. Stunkard and McLaren-Hume of the leading diets over a period of 35 years conclusively proved their failure in 9 out of 10 cases! The weight control clubs fare no better.

Dr. Walter Bloom said, in further remarks made at the symposium, that it was ". . . imperative that diet never be discussed unless there is a comparable discussion of the problem of muscular activity, physical fitness, and energy expenditure." By the same token, any discussion of physical activity—*any* exercise system—which ignores proper nutrition is likewise guilty of dealing in half measures: an impossible condition in attempting to achieve a more Vital Balance in the human body.

Setting the Record Straight

DIETS are available, quite literally, by the hundreds—and which to choose from presents no minor dilemma for the person without any special knowledge in nutrition. It is especially confusing because the subject is so larded with partial truths and distortions of the truth. Many medically sound diet concepts are borrowed in part and presented with new names and all manner of outlandish claims for quick and easy results. Often they are sugarcoated by variations on the very tiresome and totally unfounded theme that calories do not count. The low-energy diet has often been the victim of such distortion, most lately in the guise of the low-carbohydrate diet which advises the dieter to enjoy alcoholic beverages and consume all of the fats he or she craves. Clinical evaluations of this diet clearly show that any weight losses experienced are from overall caloric reduction, water loss in the system, or both.

Adding alcohol to the diet is ridiculous, and anyone performing vigorous exercise should know that *it* and alcohol do not mix. Alcoholic beverages constrict the arteries leading to the heart. When you begin exerting yourself, the heart demands a greatly accelerated blood flow. The result can be disastrous, and that goes for any vigorous activity, whether for exercise or not. The runner who has had a few drinks should allow an interval of at least two and a half hours to pass before he takes a workout.

As for a water loss in the system, we do not want any part of it. This is of particular interest to the aerobic exerciser. Running has an extremely high, continuous energy burn-off rate. Its most conspicuous accompaniment is the loss of body fluids through perspiration. This flushing out process is a healthy and a necessary one, but the system requires a replacement of these fluids. The fluid needs of the healthy body are quite astonishing until one is reminded that water makes up two-thirds of the entire bodyweight. No one could remain alive for more than several days without it. Those diets which dry out the tissues to produce weight loss are as deceptive and as damaging as the class of drugs known as the diuretics when used for weight reduction purposes. These "body blotters" which dehydrate the system are a menace to health and no aid in the conquest of the overweight condition. Such treatment is in direct contradiction to sound medical practice. *Lots of fluid is the rule to maintain good health during a reducing diet:* black coffee, tea, and water in liberal and constant dosage.

Many people do not find such fluids flavorful and are inclined to neglect a sufficient daily intake, at least six to seven glasses. The aerobic runner's body demands even more. The dieting runner has an additional obligation to attend to his fluid needs. This is the reason that, as the aerobic dieter will soon discover, soups play so important a role in the Energy-Control Diet.

Special E/C Diet Sections

The E/C Diet Planner, pages 156-157

The key to the E/C Diet, for "all Plussers," and the Diet Planner shows you how to make choices from the E/C menus. A complete daily controlled energy meal pattern for both the Fitness Dieter (FD) and the Reducing Dieter (RD).

The E/C Mealmaker Menu Section, pages 161-163
The E/C Mealmaker Recipe Section, pages 164-168

The controlled energy main dishes—nourishing, delectable, with lasting appetite satisfaction. The cornerstones of the E/C Mealmaker Menu Section.

Soup: An E/C Diet Support Food, pages 179-188

A wonderful approach to diet and a healthful precaution against dehydration of body tissues. Highly nutritious, tasty, and filling controlled energy soups. To support the main dish for complete meals. To support the diet in substituting for meals. To support the appetite between meals.

Salad: An E/C Diet Support, pages 174-178

Delicious energy control greens and garden vegetables to supply necessary vitamins, nutrients, and roughage essential to the dieter's well-being. To support the main dish for complete meals. To support the diet in substituting for meals. To support the appetite between meals.

Appetite Support Snacks, pages 188-189

Really an emergency list to choose from to support your appetite "addiction." When the craving comes on, here are the "munchers." They *will* pacify the craving which is part of a reflex chain. You bite, taste, salivate, and the hunger pangs immediately stop. Try it and see. Besides, you can enjoy tasting a lot of these negligible-calorie foods, and they are healthful as well.

Fitness & Reducing Breakfast Menus, pages 158-160
Solve the problem at a glance.

Family Fitness Recipe Section, pages 169-173
For the rapidly growing number of entire families of aerobic exercisers, here are delicious and nutritious main dish recipes for Mom, Dad, and the kids.

The Diet for All "Plussers"

THE READER will find FD and RD designations throughout the diet section. This unique feature has been introduced so that the E/C Diet may be used as a Fitness Diet by the 0+ or as a Reducing Diet by the 6+ and 16+ candidates. Recipes have been adjusted for further calorie reductions where the RD symbol appears. All recipes, both FD and RD, are energy controlled.

The FD/RD menu and recipe arrangement allows the reduced dieter to readjust his meal pattern to the FD, or maintenance level.

The FD/RD substitutive ingredients permit the mealmaker to prepare the *same dishes*, with slight adjustments, to suit both FD and RD eaters.

Control Your Weight Loss

THIS IS CERTAIN to be a diet unlike any you have been on before. May I make a prediction? You will enjoy it every bit as much or more than your regular meals! If you've heard that running makes your taste-sense keener, you're right. But you will find the recipes wonderfully flavored and seasoned, and there is lots of eating on the menus. None of the between-meals stomach-gnawing of many diets. We definitely do not want your appetite to feel deprivation. This increases cravings and eventually destroys the diet pattern. The E/C support foods are available to you just to be certain that does *not* happen. The Soup Support Section (pages 179-188) is a revelation! Soups are the diet dish par excellence! Its advantages: considerable variety, taste delectation, a sensation of fullness after eating, excellent nutritional value, limited caloric value, assured body tissue hydration.

This is not, by any stretch of the imagination, a blanket endorsement for all soups. The E/C soup recipes fulfill the dietwise specifications. They are soups for all occasions, from many ethnic backgrounds, in many flavors and consistencies. And you will be pleasantly surprised that even our impressive, hearty soup recipes, such as Minestrone and Sopa Con Albondigas (Mexican Meatball Soup), are low in calories. The soup is the ideal dietary support food. With it, it becomes a simple matter to pass up the bulky sandwich, the hurried businessman's lunch, and harried housewife's brunch.

The Energy-Control Diet is well balanced, nutritionally adequate in milk products, meat and greens, and sufficient carbohydrates to supply the important B vitamins to maintain good health. It is plenteous in protein, minerals, and vitamins as well as low in calories.

There is something else about the E/C Diet that you will enjoy. It is, where my runners are concerned, a dream diet because they do not have to go through any pencil-and-paper figuring, any splitting of hairs about food choices. I am definitely *not* implying by that that calories don't count. They do indeed, in every tiny morsel. But the leeway is considerable in the E/C Diet because:

- The recipes and various foods are energy controlled . . .

- ... within a low-energy *menu plan* (Main Dish + Support Foods) that give a double control ...

- ... plus the further RD and RD substitute ingredients control.

And in the event you are forgetting—this only accounts for *one half of the energy control*, the food intake. If you have never been on a combined diet *and* aerobic exercise program, then you are in for quite a pleasant surprise.

And a caution is in order if you are on an RD or RD+ diet: KEEP YOUR WEIGHT LOSS TO TWO POUNDS PER WEEK. If it begins to drop any faster, add a main dish meal or have enough support foods to keep your weight loss gradual. The slow loss is even more important than usual, in several respects. This time you are not acting upon your body's stored energy by diet alone. With regular aerobic exercise, there are bound to be changes *within* your system which require time to make a healthy adjustment. The weight loss will not be so superficial as by diet alone.

How to Use the E/C Reducing Diet

1. Set a Goal*

Are you a 0, 6, or 16 Plusser? Check the weight scales on page 191 according to bodyweight. Now, put down your weight loss goal. Probably, like most overweights, you've been through this routine many a time. Keep in mind that this is an entirely new ball game! Manipulating food intake with diet alone gave you none of the E/C Diet advantages. Here you have three, all working for you at the same time:

- The E/C Diet reduces the energy level of your food intake.

- Aerobic running hikes up your energy expenditure (converting your fat deposits).

- Running triggers a *new* Vital Balance to adjust your appestat control.

2. Select an E/C Diet Plan

The Energy-Control Diet Planner on page 156 is your guide to the E/C Diet. It is especially prepared to correlate to your aerobic running days and in-between days.

3. Personalize Your E/C Diet

The more you personalize your diet and apply it to your eating habits and normal routine, the more certain you are of permanent success. See "Your Eating Habitracker" on page 147. Don't be satisfied until you can arrive at the very best the E/C Diet can offer *you* to make your mealtime the happiest of experiences. Satisfy your tastes and emotional approach to eating as you attend to your overweight problem.

4. Stabilize Your Weight After Each Five-Pound Weight Loss

Go from RD to FD, add support foods as necessary. Maintain weight for one week or more before resuming weight loss as needed. (Don't lose more than two pounds per week.)

* The longer you have been overweight, the more gradual should be your weight reduction. Do not exceed two pounds weight loss per week.

Your Eating Habitracker

WE ARE ALL a collection of well-organized habits of which we are hardly aware, as psychologist William James has said. And our eating habits are certainly among the most automatic. Our appetites are conditioned according to the time of day, the places we are at, the situations we are in, and so on. To undertake a diet and apply it with a disregard, intentional or not, of our established ways, whys, and whens, of eating, as well as *what* we eat, means to act against ourselves and perhaps the most powerful of all human drives, the craving for food. This is not necessary. We can work *with* our established eating habits and more easily and painlessly change them or support them as we choose. Self-control is the word, and it underlies the entire Aerobic Fitness Program, both the running exercise and the E/C Diet.

By thinking about and making conscious your acts of eating, your appetite cravings, and when and where they occur over the course of a typical week's activity, you will have all of the information you require to truly personalize your diet plan.

Here are some of the questions you ask yourself and some of the things to look for. You can make note of this on the Eating Habitracker Profile on pages 149-155 and then use this to help you personalize your E/C Diet.

Is breakfast an important meal to you, or can you take it or leave it?

Have you always started the day with a big breakfast and if you miss it, feel a "midmorning sag"?

Which do you consider your most important meal and at what time of day do you have it?

Can you identify "the low periods" of your day which repeatedly call for appetite support, the "consolation" of "coffee and" or a candy bar?

Which are your active workdays when you put out a lot more energy and which are your most inactive?

Which days do you tend to overeat—is it on weekends? You will find that you follow a definite pattern, and

147

you must consider this in making up your E/C Diet Planner.

Are there some repeatedly uncomfortable situations, boring periods of the day which bring appetite consolation into play for you? With the great flexibility of the E/C Diet and the inspirational idea of the support foods, you can plan a menu to gain the edge on appetite and keep down the accumulation of extra pounds. What are your particular *appetite traps?* Is there some part of the midmorning that leads you to the refrigerator door—or, if you are on the job, down to the coffee shop?

Maybe your big appetite hang-up is the goggle box in the hours after work, when you flop down on the couch and eat and eat? Research has shown that late evenings, as a general rule, are the time when those with overweight problems do most of their eating. Up to 800 calories' worth! And most of it unconscious. This is what is called *automatic eating,* and observing yourself will reveal it—a first step in bringing eating under self-control. Incidentally, this late-hour overeating is referred to by psychiatrists as the "night-eating syndrome."

Track those habits and you'll be bound to make some surprising discoveries. One of my runners, a woman of forty-four and a real estate broker, found that she was getting up to eat something each time a food or drink commercial came on her television set! Like the famous experiment with the Pavlov dog, she was salivating at the *image* of food. This would be called her conditioned reflex. We all have such eating habits, and once they become conscious, they *can* be controlled. But not by immediate denial. Better to support the habit with low-energy snacks and then gently change it if you wish to.

Ask yourself the question when you begin to eat—"Am I hungry?" And ask it halfway through your meal. See how your leftover portions begin to grow. This will tell you that you are eating for taste rather than hunger. And as soon as the taste novelty of the food is gone, you can quit it instead of consuming the rest by habit alone.

Eating Habitracker Profile

Tracking your Eating Habits: For one typical week, keep a daily record of your eating patterns. Make note of meals, large, moderate or small; between-meal snacks; periods of appetite craving, "appetite traps" which lead to eating. For suggestions of what to pay special attention to, see page 147.

MONDAY:

Breakfast _____

_____

Lunch _____

_____

Dinner _____

_____

Late Evening _____

_____

Between Meals _____

_____

_____

Appetite Traps _____

_____

_____

TUESDAY:

Breakfast _____

_____

_____

Lunch _____

_____

_____

Dinner _____

_____

_____

Late Evening _____

_____

_____

Between Meals _____

_____

_____

Appetite Traps _____

_____

_____

WEDNESDAY:

Breakfast_____

_____

_____

Lunch_____

_____

_____

Dinner_____

_____

_____

Late Evening_____

_____

_____

Between Meals_____

_____

_____

Appetite Traps_____

_____

_____

THURSDAY:

Breakfast_____

_____

_____

Lunch_____

_____

_____

Dinner_____

_____

_____

Late Evening_____

_____

_____

Between Meals_____

_____

_____

Appetite Traps_____

_____

_____

FRIDAY:

Breakfast_____

_____

_____

Lunch_____

_____

_____

Dinner_____

_____

_____

Late Evening_____

_____

_____

Between Meals_____

_____

_____

Appetite Traps_____

_____

_____

SATURDAY:

Breakfast _____

_____

_____

Lunch _____

_____

_____

Dinner _____

_____

_____

Late Evening _____

_____

_____

Between Meals _____

_____

_____

Appetite Traps _____

_____

_____

SUNDAY:

Breakfast _____

_____

_____

Lunch _____

_____

_____

Dinner _____

_____

_____

Late Evening _____

_____

_____

Between Meals _____

_____

_____

Appetite Traps _____

_____

_____

ENERGY-CONTROL

This is the guide to your E/C Diet. Whether you are 0+, 6+, or 16+—pick your appropriate column and choose a diet pattern. Your next step is the E/C menus for breakfast and maindish meals

	Daily On 3 Running Days
0+ All FD choices except as otherwise noted; can switch to RD if weight change warrants.	FD Breakfast 2 FD Mealmaker Menus* Limit 2 Salads with Mealmaker Menus or as Appetite Support during day Limit 2 Soups with Mealmaker Menus or as Appetite Support during day Appetite Snack Supports * May wish to reduce to 1, but running exercise burns lots of energy and adjusts appestat.
6+ 6% to 11% FD or RD, according to desired weight loss. 12% to 16% RD only	FD or RD Breakfast 1 FD or RD Mealmaker Menu Limit 2 Salads 1 Mealmaker Menu replacement, 1 with Mealmaker Menu or as Appetite Support during day Limit 2 Soups 1 Mealmaker Menu replacement, 1 with Mealmaker Menu or as Appetite Support during day Appetite Snack Supports
16+ RD only	RD Breakfast 1 RD Mealmaker Menu Limit 2 Soups 1 Mealmaker Menu replacement, 1 with Mealmaker Menu or as Appetite Support during day Limit 1 Salad 1 with Mealmaker Menu or as Appetite Support during day Appetite Snack Supports

DIET PLANNER

(The Mealmaker Menus). The menus mark those special dishes for which E/C recipes are supplied in the appropriate sections.

Daily Between Running Days	Soupfest* Saladfest*

FD Breakfast
2 Mealmaker Menus—1 FD, 1 RD
Limit 2 Salads
  with Mealmaker Menus or as
  Appetite Support during day
Limit 2 Soups
  with Mealmaker Menus or as
  Appetite Support during day
Appetite Snack Supports	

RD Breakfast
1 RD Mealmaker Menu
Limit 2 Salads
  1 Mealmaker Menu replacement,
  1 with Mealmaker Menu or
  as Appetite Support during day
Limit 2 Soups
  1 with Mealmaker Menu,
  1 as Appetite Support during
  day or Mealmaker Menu
  replacement
Appetite Snack Supports
	1 FD Breakfast
	2 Soups
	  1 meal replacement,
	  1 Appetite Support
	  during day
	2 Salads
	  1 meal replacement,
	  1 Appetite Support
	  during day
	Appetite Snack Supports

RD Breakfast
1 Soup
1 Salad
1 RD Mealmaker Menu
Appetite Snack Supports
	1 RD Breakfast
	1 Soup or Salad
	  meal replacement
	1 Soup or Salad
	  meal replacement
	Appetite Snack Supports
	* For additional weight loss, use
	Soup Day or Salad Day menus
	above for 1 or 2 days of the
	week. Recommended for 12-
	16%, prescribed for 16+.

Energy-Control Breakfast Menus

Fitness Diet (FD)
Reducing Diet (RD)

FD

Orange juice . . . . ½ cup
Wheat flakes . . . .
   with small sliced banana
   or 1 cup sliced fresh peaches
   and 1 cup milk
Toast . . . . 2 slices, enriched bread
Butter . . . . 2 teaspoons
Coffee or tea*

RD

Orange juice . . . . ½ cup
Wheat flakes . . . . 1 cup
   with 1 cup skimmed milk
Coffee or tea†

FD

Tomato juice . . . . ½ cup
Poached eggs 2
Crisp bacon . . . . 2 strips
Whole wheat toast . . . . 1 slice
Butter . . . . 1 teaspoon
Marmalade, jelly, or jam . . . . . 1 teaspoon
Milk . . . . 1 cup
Coffee or tea*

RD

Tomato juice . . . . ½ cup
Poached egg 1
Crisp bacon . . . . 2 strips
   or Whole wheat toast . . . . . 1 slice
   with 1 teaspoon butter or 2
   teaspoons dietetic margarine
Skimmed milk . . . . 1 cup
Coffee or tea†

* = If desired, with cream (1 tablespoon) and sugar (1 teaspoon).
† = No cream or sugar. If desired, use artificial sweetener and a slice
of lemon with the tea.

FD

Grapefruit half
French toast . . . . 2 slices, made with
enriched bread, ½ egg,
and milk
Butter. . . . . 2 teaspoons
Jelly, jam, or preserves . . . . . 2 tablespoons
Milk . . . . 1 cup
Coffee or tea*

RD

Grapefruit half
French toast . . . . 1 slice, made with enriched
bread, ½ egg, and milk
Butter. . . . . 1 teaspoon, or 2 teaspoons
dietetic margarine
Jelly, jam, or preserves . . . . . 1½ teaspoons
Skimmed milk . . . . 1 cup
Coffee or tea†

FD

Cantaloupe half
Omelet . . . . made with 1 large egg
Grilled ham . . . . 2 ounces
Whole wheat toast . . . . 2 slices
Butter. . . . . 2 teaspoons
Milk . . . . 1 cup
Coffee or tea*

RD

Cantaloupe half
Omelet . . . . made with 1 large egg
Whole wheat toast . . . . 1 slice
Butter. . . . . 1 teaspoon, or 2 teaspoons
dietetic margarine
Skimmed milk . . . . 1 cup
Coffee or tea†

* = If desired, with cream (1 tablespoon) and sugar (1 teaspoon).
† = No cream or sugar. If desired, use artificial sweetener and a slice
of lemon with the tea.

FD

Fresh strawberries . . . . 1 cup
   with 1 teaspoon sugar
Oatmeal . . . . 1 cup
   with 1 cup milk
Toast . . . . 2 slices, enriched bread
Butter . . . . 2 teaspoons
Marmalade, jelly, or jam . . . . . 2 teaspoons
Coffee or tea*

RD

Fresh strawberries . . . . 1 cup
   with artificial sweetener to taste
Oatmeal . . . . ¾ cup
   with 1 cup skimmed milk
Toast . . . . 1 slice, enriched bread
Butter . . . . 1 teaspoon, or 2 teaspoons
                           dietetic margarine

Coffee or tea†

FD

Orange juice . . . . ½ cup
Soft-boiled egg 1
Crisp bacon . . . . 2 strips
Whole wheat toast . . . . 2 slices
Butter . . . . 2 teaspoons
Milk . . . . 1 cup
Coffee or tea*

RD

Orange juice . . . . ½ cup
Soft-boiled egg 1
Whole wheat toast . . . . 1 slice
Butter . . . . 1 teaspoon, or 2 teaspoons
                           dietetic margarine
Skimmed milk . . . . 1 cup
Coffee or tea†

* = If desired, with cream (1 tablespoon) and sugar (1 teaspoon).
† = No cream or sugar. If desired, use artificial sweetener and a slice of lemon with the tea.

Energy-Control Mealmaker Menus

Broiled lobster*
Small baked potato (FD)
    or string beans (unlimited—RD)
Tossed green salad
    with bleu cheese dressing (FD) or bottled low-calorie
    bleu cheese dressing (RD)
Fresh strawberries: 1½ cups in 2 tablespoons sour cream
    (FD) or 1 cup in 2 tablespoons imitation sour cream
    (RD)
Coffee or tea†

Lamb chop New Orleans*
Orange and onion salad*—1 serving
Mashed potatoes: ⅔ cup (FD) or ⅓ cup (RD)
Ice cream (1 individual contained—FD) or Jell-O (½ cup—
    RD)
Coffee or tea†

Herb-baked chicken*
Molded pear salad*—1 serving
Broccoli spears: 1½ cups (FD) or ¾ cup (RD)
Iced cupcake (FD) or dietetic chocolate pudding (1 serv-
    ing—RD)
Coffee or tea†

A Danish hamburger*
Sliced tomatoes, sprinkled with dill: 2 large (FD) or 2
    small (RD)
Asparagus spears: 12 (FD) or 6 (RD)
Fresh fruit cup
Coffee or tea†

Fish kebab*
Fluffy boiled rice: ⅔ cup (FD) or ⅓ cup (RD)
Spinach, with lemon wedge: 1½ cups (FD) or ¾ cup (RD)
Canned apricot halves: 8 medium with 4 tablespoons syrup
    (FD) or 4 medium with 2 tablespoons syrup (RD)
Coffee or tea†

* = Recipe included in this volume.
† = For RD, use artificial sweetener and no cream.

Tomato or V-8 vegetable juice: 1 cup (FD) or ½ cup (RD)
Mixed English grill*
Tossed green salad with Italian dressing (FD) or bottled
    low-calorie Italian dressing (RD)
Cantaloupe half
Coffee or tea†

Lemon-broiled chicken*
Cole slaw, French-style*—1 serving
Green peas with tiny onions: 1 cup (FD) or ½ cup (RD)
Rice pudding (½ cup—FD) or Sliced banana, 1 medium, in
    ¼ cup skimmed milk (RD)
Coffee or tea†

Steak Tartare*
Gala salad bowl*—1 serving
Diced beets: 1⅓ cups (FD) or ⅔ cup (RD)
Angel food cake (1 small wedge—FD) or grapefruit half
    (RD)
Coffee or tea†

Sweetbreads en brochette*
Fluffy boiled rice: ½ cup (FD) or ¼ cup (RD)
Belgian endive salad*—1 serving
Carrots: 1½ cups (FD) or ¾ cup (RD)
Fresh raspberries: 1 cup with ¼ cup milk (FD) or ¼ cup
    skimmed milk (RD)
Coffee or tea†

Barbecued cod*
1 small baked or boiled potato
Brussels sprouts: 1½ cups (FD) or ¾ cup (RD)
Cucumber salad with chervil*—1 serving
Pumpkin or custard pie (4-inch piece—FD) or 1 tangerine
    (RD)
Coffee or tea†

Herbed beef on rye*
Relishes: Celery and carrot sticks, radishes, scallions, a small
    dill pickle, and 3 large green olives
String beans (unlimited)
Stewed tomatoes: 1 cup (FD) or ½ cup (RD)
Apple snow (1 cup—FD) or 1 small apple (RD)
Coffee or tea†

* = Recipe included in this volume.
† = For RD, use artificial sweetener and no cream.

Tomato soup (½ cup—FD) or consommé (½ cup—RD)
Shish kebab*
Rice pilaf (FD only—½ cup)
Persian cucumber yogurt salad*—1 serving
Sherbet (½ cup—FD) or a small bunch of seedless grapes
    (RD)
Coffee or tea†

* = Recipe included in this volume.
† = For RD, use artificial sweetener and no cream.

Energy-Control Mealmaker Recipes*

BROILED LOBSTER

1 small lobster (about 1 pound)   Salt and pepper
1 teaspoon melted butter (FD)   Lemon wedge
   or dietetic margarine (RD)

Have your fish dealer clean, split, and prepare the lobster for cooking. (Lobsters must be cooked very soon after killing.) Place on broiler rack, shell side down. Brush with melted butter or margarine. Broil slowly until meat is browned—about 15 minutes. Sprinkle with salt and pepper. Serve with lemon wedge.

LAMB CHOP NEW ORLEANS

1 lamb shoulder chop,   1 tablespoon finely chopped
   ½-inch thick   green pepper
1 teaspoon butter (FD) or   1 tablespoon finely chopped
   dietetic margarine (RD)   onion
Salt and pepper   Pinch of garlic powder
½ cup tomato juice   Pinch of rosemary

Brown chop on both sides in butter or margarine. Season to taste with salt and pepper. Add remaining ingredients. Cover and simmer until meat is tender.

HERB-BAKED CHICKEN

1 chicken thigh and   Basil or thyme
   1 drumstick   Salt
1 tablespoon garlic French   Pepper
   dressing (FD) or low-
   calorie dressing (RD)

Tear off a piece of aluminum foil large enough to enclose the chicken. Place chicken on foil. Brush with dressing. Sprinkle with basil or thyme and salt and pepper. Wrap foil around chicken and refrigerate for 1 hour. Bake in preheated 350° oven until done.

Variation: Place a thick slice of onion on top of chicken before enclosing in foil.

* One-portion servings.

A DANISH HAMBURGER

¼ pound ground lean beef
1 egg
Salt and pepper to taste
1 ounce Danish bleu cheese
2 teaspoons softened butter
    (FD) or dietetic margarine
    (RD)

½ teaspoon Worcestershire
    sauce
⅛ teaspoon dry mustard
¼ teaspoon minced fresh
    parsley
Drop of lemon juice

Combine ground beef, egg, salt and pepper and mix well. With a fork, mash together the bleu cheese, butter or margarine, Worcestershire sauce, mustard, parsley, and lemon juice. Shape the beef into two thin patties. Spoon bleu cheese mixture onto one of the patties. Top with remaining patty, sealing the edges together. Broil in preheated broiler, 4 inches from heat, to desired doneness.

FISH KEBAB

1 fillet of sole or halibut
    (about ¼ pound)
Salt, white pepper, and paprika
2 tiny whole onions, parboiled
2 cherry tomatoes
2 mushroom caps

2 pimiento-stuffed green olives
2 teaspoons butter (FD) or
    dietetic margarine (RD),
    melted
1 teaspoon lemon juice

Sprinkle fish with salt, pepper and paprika. Fold in half, lengthwise, and place on a skewer, along with the onions, cherry tomatoes, mushroom caps, and olives. Combine melted butter or margarine with lemon juice. Place kebab on greased broiler rack and brush with the lemon butter. Broil for about 5 minutes, 3 inches from the heat. Turn, brush with remaining lemon butter, and broil until fish flakes when tested with a fork.

MIXED ENGLISH GRILL

½ veal kidney
1 teaspoon vinegar
1 tablespoon butter (FD) or
    dietetic margarine (RD)
1 tablespoon lemon juice
1 teaspoon minced fresh parsley
Salt and pepper to taste
Dash paprika
2 teaspoons melted butter (FD)
    or dietetic margarine (RD)

1 tablespoon bread crumbs
Pinch each of basil and
    rosemary
2 slices bacon
2 link sausages (FD only)
1 loin lamb chop (FD only)
1 tomato, halved
1 individual steak
Chopped fresh parsley

Place veal kidney in saucepan with 1 cup water and the vinegar. Bring to a boil. Lower heat, cover, and simmer for about 10 minutes. Drain, cover, and refrigerate.

To make butter sauce: Melt the butter and add lemon juice, parsley, salt, pepper, and paprika. To make crumb topping: Combine bread crumbs with melted butter, basil, and rosemary.

Fry bacon until crisp and drain on paper towels; keep warm. Place sausages in a skillet with cold water to cover and bring to boil. Drain, cook until browned, then set aside and keep warm.

Place lamb chop on broiler rack. Brush with some of the butter sauce. Broil to desired doneness on one side, 6 inches from the heat. Turn chop, arrange tomato halves, cut side up, on broiler rack. Brush chop and tomato with butter sauce. Broil for about 10 minutes.

Pan-fry the steak to desired doneness, brushing with butter sauce before and after turning. Keep warm.

Spoon crumb topping over tomato halves. Remove chop and keep warm. Arrange kidney, cut side up, on broiler rack. Brush with butter sauce. Broil kidney and tomato until crumbs are golden—about 2 minutes.

Arrange bacon, sausages, steak, chop, kidney and tomato on platter. Sprinkle with chopped fresh parsley.

LEMON-BROILED CHICKEN

½ broiler	2 tablespoons melted butter
½ lemon	(FD) or dietetic margarine
Salt and pepper	(RD)
Paprika	1 teaspoon minced fresh parsley
	1 teaspoon minced chives

Rub the surface of the chicken with cut side of lemon, squeezing out the juice. Sprinkle with salt, pepper, and paprika. Place chicken, skin side down, on greased broiler rack. Combine melted butter or margarine, parsley, and chives. Brush top side of chicken with some of the butter mixture. Broil 3 or 4 inches from the flame for 12 to 15 minutes. Turn chicken and brush again with butter mixture. Continue broiling until done, basting frequently with butter mixture.

STEAK TARTARE

¼ pound ground sirloin
1 teaspoon grated onion
Pinch of garlic powder
1 teaspoon minced parsley
Dash Worcestershire sauce
Pinch of dry mustard

Salt and pepper to taste
1 raw egg yolk
1 slice of rye or pumpernickel
    bread (FD) or protein
    bread (RD), toasted

Combine the ground sirloin with onion, garlic powder, parsley, Worcestershire sauce, dry mustard, and salt and pepper. Mound onto a slice of toast. Make a depression in the center of the meat, and drop in the egg yolk.

SWEETBREADS EN BROCHETTE

¼ pound sweetbreads
1 slice bacon
Salt and pepper

1 teaspoon butter (FD) or
    dietetic margarine (RD),
    melted

Cover sweetbreads with water and simmer for 20 minutes. Drain well and cut into 1-inch cubes. Cut the bacon into 1-inch pieces. Alternate sweetbread cubes and bacon pieces on skewer. Brush with melted butter or margarine. Broil slowly until bacon is crisp—about 10 minutes—turning to brown evenly.

BARBECUED COD

¼ pound cod
Salt to taste
¼ cup tomato catsup
2 teaspoons lemon juice
½ teaspoon vinegar
2 teaspoons butter (FD) or
    dietetic margarine (RD)

1 teaspoon honey (or artificial
    sweetener to taste for RD)
1 tablespoon minced onion
½ teaspoon minced parsley
¼ teaspoon Worcestershire
    sauce
Dash Tabasco

Place the fish in a greased baking dish, skin side down, and sprinkle with salt. Combine the remaining ingredients in a small saucepan, and heat to the boiling point. Spread sauce thinly over the fish. Broil under moderate heat until fish flakes when tested with a fork—about 15 minutes. Baste with sauce every few minutes.

HERBED BEEF ON RYE

¼ pound ground lean beef
⅛ teaspoon basil
1 teaspoon chopped fresh
   parsley

Salt and pepper to taste
1 egg
1 tablespoon milk
1 slice rye bread, lightly toasted

Combine ground beef with basil, parsley, salt and pepper. Add egg and milk and mix thoroughly. Spoon beef mixture onto toasted rye bread, spreading evenly to the edge. Broil to desired doneness.

SHISH KEBAB

¼ pound lean lamb,
   cut into cubes
1 tablespoon safflower oil
1 tablespoon lemon juice
1 tablespoon orange juice
1 tablespoon dry red wine
Salt, pepper, and garlic powder
   to taste

Pinch each of oregano and
   thyme
4 tiny whole onions
1 tomato, halved,
   or 4 cherry tomatoes
Chunks of green pepper
4 mushroom caps

Combine oil, lemon juice, orange juice, wine, salt, pepper, garlic powder, oregano, and thyme. Place lamb cubes into marinade and refrigerate for several hours, turning occasionally. Arrange marinated lamb cubes and vegetables on a skewer. Brush with the marinade. Broil 3 inches from the heat to desired doneness, turning to cook evenly.

Energy-Control Family Fitness Recipes

HERBED RIB ROAST OF BEEF

5-pound standing rib roast of beef
1 clove garlic, cut into thin slivers
1 teaspoon salt
½ teaspoon dried marjoram
¼ teaspoon black pepper

Place meat in shallow roasting pan, fat side up. Cut slits in fat on top of the roast and insert a garlic sliver in each slit. Combine salt, marjoram, and pepper, and rub the mixture into sides and top of roast. Roast, uncovered, in 325° oven to desired doneness—about 2 hours for medium-rare beef.

SPICED POT ROAST

5-pound chuck roast
2 tablespoons safflower oil
2 cups tomato juice
1 tablespoon wine vinegar
1 cup chopped onions
1 clove garlic, crushed
1 bay leaf, crumbled
2 teaspoons cinnamon
2 teaspoons ginger
2 teaspoons salt
¼ teaspoon pepper
1 tablespoon sugar (FD) or equivalent of artificial sweetener (RD)
2 teaspoons minced parsley

In a large, heavy pan, brown the meat on all sides in oil. Combine the remaining ingredients, mix well, and pour over the meat. Cover and simmer until the meat is tender—about 4 hours. Makes 6 servings.

LAMB STEW

2 pounds stewing lamb, cubed
Flour
Butter or cooking oil (FD) or dietetic margarine (RD)
3 cups tomato juice
1 clove garlic
2 teaspoons celery seeds
Salt to taste
4 peppercorns
4 carrots, pared and quartered
6 small white onions, halved
4 sprigs parsley
2 teaspoons Worcestershire sauce
Chopped fresh parsley

Lightly grease pan with butter, margarine, or oil. Roll lamb cubes in flour, and brown well on all sides. Add tomato juice, garlic, celery seeds, salt, peppercorns, carrots, onions, parsley sprigs, and Worcestershire sauce. Cover and simmer until lamb is fork-tender. Garnish with chopped fresh parsley. Makes 6 to 8 servings.

POACHED CHICKEN

4-pound chicken
Boiling water
1 onion, sliced
1 carrot, cut up
2 sprigs thyme

1 bay leaf
2 teaspoons salt
A few peppercorns
2 sprigs parsley
1 whole onion, peeled

Have the chicken cleaned and prepared as for roasting. Put the parsley sprigs and whole onion in the cavity. Sew the opening securely and truss. Place the chicken in a deep kettle, and add boiling water to cover. Add the sliced onion, carrot, thyme, bay leaf, and peppercorns. Cover and simmer gently until tender—about 2 hours. Add salt during last hour of cooking. Transfer the chicken to serving platter and serve the broth as the first course. Makes 4 servings.

HUNGARIAN GOULASH

2 pounds top round, cut in
    1-inch cubes
1 cup tomato juice
1 cup consommé
1 small green pepper, diced
2 cloves garlic
1 teaspoon Hungarian paprika

¾ teaspoon salt
½ teaspoon pepper
1 small bay leaf
6 small carrots, cut in 1-inch
    pieces
Chopped fresh parsley

Place the meat in a large, heavy pot. Add tomato juice, consommé, green pepper, garlic, paprika, salt, pepper, and bay leaf. Cover and simmer for 2½ hours. Add carrots and continue cooking until meat and carrots are tender. Garnish with chopped fresh parsley. Makes 6 servings.

SAVORY MEAT LOAF

1 pound lean ground beef
1 egg
½ cup soft bread crumbs
    (RD, use protein bread)
½ cup milk (FD) or skimmed
    milk (RD)
2 tablespoons minced fresh
    parsley
2 tablespoons grated onion

1 clove garlic, minced
¼ teaspoon basil
¼ teaspoon oregano
⅛ teaspoon rosemary
Pinch of thyme
¼ teaspoon paprika
Salt and pepper to taste
2 slices bacon

Soak the bread crumbs in milk and add to ground beef. Add the egg, parsley, garlic, onion, and seasonings. Mix well. Shape into a loaf or pat into a loaf pan. Place the bacon slices on top. Bake in 350° oven until meat loaf is done—about 1 hour. Serve hot or cold. Makes 4 servings.

ROAST LEG OF LAMB WITH ARTICHOKES

5-pound leg of lamb	2 cloves garlic, cut into slivers
2 teaspoons salt	4 small artichokes
¼ teaspoon pepper	1 tablespoon white wine vinegar
1 teaspoon rosemary	3 tablespoons lemon juice

Have your butcher prepare the lamb for roasting.

Combine the salt, pepper, and rosemary. Make several slits in the lamb. Rub outside of meat with the salt mixture, and insert garlic slivers in the slits. Place meat on a rack in roasting pan. Roast in preheated 425° oven for half an hour or until meat is nicely browned. Reduce heat to 325°, and continue roasting for another hour.

Remove the tough outer leaves of the artichokes and cut off the stems. Cut artichokes in half lengthwise and scoop out the choke. Place in boiling salted water, add vinegar, and simmer until just tender—about half an hour. Drain. Place the artichoke halves in roasting pan around the lamb. Pour the lemon juice over the meat, sprinkling a little on the artichokes. Cover pan and roast 15 minutes longer. Makes 4 servings.

BAKED HADDOCK

1 pound haddock fillets, fresh or frozen	2 teaspoons minced onion
2 tablespoons butter (FD) or dietetic margarine (RD), melted	½ teaspoon salt
	⅛ teaspoon pepper
	Pinch of paprika
1 tablespoon lemon juice	Chopped fresh parsley

If using frozen fish, thaw according to package instructions. Place the fillets in a greased shallow baking dish. Combine the melted butter or margarine, lemon juice, onion, salt, pepper, and paprika. Pour over the fish. Bake in a 400° oven until fish flakes when tested with a fork. Garnish with a sprinkling of chopped fresh parsley. Makes 4 servings.

PORK CHOPS CALIFORNIA

6 loin pork chops, fat trimmed
off
Butter (FD) or dietetic
margarine (RD)
1 medium onion, chopped
6 tablespoons chili sauce
1 clove garlic

3 tablespoons lemon juice
½ teaspoon dry mustard
2 teaspoons sugar (FD) or
equivalent of artificial
sweetener (RD)
1 teaspoon Worcestershire sauce
Salt and pepper to taste

Combine the chopped onion, chili sauce, garlic, lemon juice, sugar, Worcestershire sauce, dry mustard, salt, and pepper. Pour over the chops and let stand 1 hour. Melt some butter or margarine in a heavy skillet. Drain the chops, reserving sauce, and brown on both sides. Add the sauce, cover, and simmer until chops are done. Makes 6 servings.

CHICKEN ESPAGÑOLE

2 to 2½ pound chicken, cut in
serving pieces
2 large tomatoes, peeled and
diced
1 green pepper, chopped
1 large onion, chopped

½ cup capers
1 cup pimiento-stuffed green
olives, sliced
1 teaspoon chili powder
1 teaspoon salt

Place all the ingredients in a pot. Add just enough water to cover. Simmer, covered, until chicken is tender. Makes 4 servings.

MEATBALLS WITH LEMON SAUCE

1½ pounds lean ground beef
2 tablespoons chopped parsley
1 clove garlic, crushed
1 small onion, finely chopped
1 teaspoon salt
¼ teaspoon pepper
¼ teaspoon oregano
3 tablespoons rice

2 cups beef bouillon
2 tablespoons flour
2 eggs
2 tablespoons lemon juice
1 tablespoon dry red wine
½ teaspoon honey
½ teaspoon grated lemon rind

Combine ground beef, parsley, garlic, onion, salt, pepper, oregano, rice, and ⅓ cup bouillon. Shape into 2-inch balls and roll in the flour. Bring the remaining bouillon to a boil. Add the meatballs and simmer, covered, until rice is tender—about 35 minutes.

Beat the eggs until light. Then beat in lemon juice, wine,

and honey. Add grated lemon rind. Gradually pour in the broth from the meatballs, and blend the mixture with a wire whisk. Return sauce to meatballs. Heat over very low flame for a few minutes, until the sauce is just thickened. Makes 6 servings.

SPICED SHANK OF BEEF

3 pounds beef shank
¼ cup wine vinegar
2 tablespoons sugar (FD) or equivalent of artificial sweetener (RD)
½ teaspoon ground cloves
½ teaspoon cinnamon
⅛ teaspoon mace
1 bay leaf, crumbled
1 teaspoon Worcestershire sauce
½ teaspoon pepper
1 large onion, sliced
2 teaspoons salt
2 tablespoons safflower oil
Hot water

Cut the meat into serving-size pieces and place in a deep bowl. Combine vinegar, sugar or artificial sweetener, cloves, cinnamon, mace, bay leaf, Worcestershire sauce, salt and pepper. Cook and stir for 5 minutes. Cool. Pour over the meat and let stand 4 hours, turning meat occasionally. Heat the oil in a large, heavy pan. Brown the meat and onion in it. Add marinade plus hot water to cover the meat. Simmer, covered, until meat is tender—about 2 hours. Strain the gravy and serve with the meat (FD only). Makes 6 servings.

Salads: An Energy-Control Support Food

GALA SALAD BOWL

1 small head Boston lettuce	½ cup thinly sliced celery
1 small head romaine	1 cucumber, pared and thinly
Chicory leaves	sliced
⅛ pound fresh spinach	6 radishes, sliced thin
1 Belgian endive	6 fresh mushrooms, sliced
½ bunch watercress	

Tear Boston lettuce, romaine, chicory, and spinach into bite-size pieces into salad bowl. Cut endive into thick crosswise slices. Add to salad bowl, along with the watercress, celery, cucumber, radishes, and mushrooms. Toss to combine. Serve with a light French (vinaigrette) dressing. For RD, use your favorite bottled low-calorie dressing. Makes 6 servings.

BELGIAN ENDIVE SALAD

8 stalks Belgian endive	2 tablespoons white wine vinegar
4 scallions, sliced	⅛ teaspoon paprika
Salt and pepper	Pinch of sugar
2 tablespoons safflower oil	Chopped fresh parsley

Place endive in ice water to crisp. Drain and dry with paper towels. Trim off root end, then cut into thick crosswise slices. Season to taste with salt and pepper, and combine with the scallions. Combine the oil, vinegar, paprika, and sugar. Pour over salad and toss gently until endive is coated. Sprinkle with chopped fresh parsley. Makes 6 servings.

COLE SLAW, FRENCH-STYLE

3 cups shredded cabbage	1 teaspoon salt
1 carrot, coarsely grated	⅛ teaspoon freshly ground
½ green pepper, finely shredded	black pepper
2 tablespoons safflower oil	¼ teaspoon celery or
2 tablespoons white wine	caraway seeds
vinegar	¼ teaspoon sugar
1 tablespoon lemon juice	⅛ teaspoon dry mustard

Combine cabbage, carrot, and green pepper in salad bowl.

Combine the remaining ingredients in a jar and shake vigorously. Pour over the vegetables and toss until they are coated. Chill. Toss the salad once again just before serving. Makes 4 to 6 servings.

PERSIAN CUCUMBER YOGURT SALAD

4 medium cucumbers, pared
and sliced thin
1½ teaspoons salt
1 clove garlic, crushed
1 tablespoon lemon juice
1 tablespoon white wine vinegar

1½ cups yogurt
1 tablespoon snipped fresh dill
1 tablespoon safflower oil
2 teaspoons chopped fresh
mint or parsley

Sprinkle cucumbers with the salt and let stand for 15 minutes. Combine garlic, lemon juice, vinegar, yogurt and dill. Mix until well blended. Add to cucumbers and toss. Sprinkle oil over the top, and garnish with chopped fresh mint or parsley. Makes 6 servings.

CAESAR SALAD

1 clove garlic
2 heads romaine
4 tablespoons olive oil (FD)
or bottled low-calorie
Italian dressing (RD)
Salt and freshly ground black
pepper to taste

1 raw egg
1 lemon, halved
6 anchovy fillets, cut in small
pieces
4 tablespoons grated Parmesan
or Romano cheese
Croutons

Rub the salad bowl with garlic clove. Tear romaine in bite-size pieces into bowl. Pour oil or bottled dressing over the romaine, sprinkle with salt and pepper, and toss until romaine is well coated. Break the egg over the romaine. Squeeze the juice from the lemon, and pour over the salad. Toss gently until well blended. Add anchovies, cheese, and croutons (only a few if RD) and toss again. Makes 6 servings.

ORANGE AND ONION SALAD

3 large oranges, peeled or
unpeeled, sliced thin
3 large Bermuda, Italian, or
Spanish onions, peeled and
sliced thin

2 tablespoons safflower oil
1 tablespoon orange juice
1 tablespoon lemon juice
Salt, pepper, and rosemary

Alternate the orange slices with onion slices on salad platter. Combine the oil, orange juice, lemon juice, salt and pepper to taste, and a pinch of rosemary. Blend well and pour over the salad. Makes 6 servings.

GREEK SALAD

1 head iceberg lettuce
1 head chicory
3 scallions, sliced, or 1 small onion, sliced and separated into rings
1 dozen Greek olives
2 ounces feta cheese, cubed
4 tablespoons olive oil*

2 tablespoons white wine vinegar†
1 tablespoon lemon juice
Salt and freshly ground black pepper to taste
⅛ teaspoon dry mustard
⅛ teaspoon paprika
1 clove garlic

Rub salad bowl with garlic clove. Tear lettuce and chicory in bitesize pieces into salad bowl. Add scallions or onion, olives, and cheese. Combine the oil, vinegar, lemon juice, salt, pepper, mustard, and paprika. Blend well. Pour over salad and toss gently until greens are coated. Makes 6 servings.

CUCUMBER SALAD WITH CHERVIL

2 large cucumbers, pared and thinly sliced
2 tablespoons safflower oil
2 tablespoons white wine vinegar

Salt and freshly ground black pepper to taste
2 teaspoons chopped fresh chervil
Watercress or escarole

Combine the oil, vinegar, salt and pepper in a jar and shake vigorously. Pour over the cucumber slices. Let stand for several hours, turning frequently, until cucumbers are wilted and mellow. Arrange on a bed of watercress or escarole. Sprinkle with chopped chervil. Makes 6 servings.

CALIFORNIA SPINACH SALAD

1 pound tender, young spinach
½ pound fresh mushrooms, sliced
1 small raw egg
¼ teaspoon salt
⅛ teaspoon dry mustard
⅛ teaspoon paprika
½ teaspoon sugar

¼ teaspoon Worcestershire sauce
½ cup tomato juice
2 tablespoons safflower oil
2 tablespoons lemon juice or wine vinegar
½ clove garlic, crushed

* For RD, substitute bottled low-calorie Italian dressing for oil and vinegar. Add lemon juice and taste for seasoning.

Place the egg, salt, mustard, paprika, sugar, Worcestershire sauce, and tomato juice in a bowl, and mix until blended. Alternately and slowly, beat in the oil and lemon juice or vinegar. Add crushed garlic.

Tear the spinach in bite-size pieces into salad bowl. Add mushrooms and toss to combine. Pour in as much dressing as is needed to moisten the vegetables. Toss. Makes 6 servings.

STUFFED TOMATO SALAD A LA RUSSE

Entrée Salad

6 large tomatoes
⅓ cup diced cucumber
⅓ cup cooked lima beans
¼ cup chopped celery
1 tablespoon capers
1 tablespoon chopped scallions
Salt and pepper
Wine vinegar or lemon juice

½ cup diced cooked shrimp, chicken, salmon, or veal
Russian dressing or mayonnaise (FD) or low-calorie mayonnaise (RD)
Crisp lettuce leaves
Chopped fresh parsley or dill

Peel the tomatoes if desired. Remove a thin slice from the top of each, and hollow out the center, reserving the pulp. Sprinkle the inside with salt, turn over, and let stand for 30 minutes to drain. Combine ⅓ cup of the reserved tomato pulp, cucumber, lima beans, celery, capers, scallions. Season to taste with salt, pepper, and vinegar or lemon juice. Add shrimp, chicken, salmon, or veal. Bind with Russian dressing or mayonnaise. Stuff the tomatoes and serve on lettuce leaves. Sprinkle with chopped fresh parsley or dill. Makes 6 servings.

ITALIAN GREEN BEAN SALAD

1 pound string beans, cut lengthwise into slivers, cooked and drained
4 tablespoons safflower oil*
3 tablespoons wine vinegar
½ teaspoon salt
¼ teaspoon freshly ground black pepper

½ clove garlic, crushed
1 teaspoon oregano, powdered between fingers
1 small red Italian onion, sliced and separated into rings
Crisp lettuce leaves

Combine the oil, vinegar, salt, pepper, and garlic in a jar and shake vigorously. Pour dressing over beans and toss. Add onion rings and oregano and toss again. Chill. Serve on crisp lettuce leaves. Makes 6 servings.

* For RD, substitute bottled low-calorie Italian dressing for the oil, vinegar, and other dressing ingredients.

MOLDED PEAR SALAD

2 envelopes raspberry-flavored Jell-O (FD) or dietetic dessert gelatin (RD)
4 canned pear halves (dietetic pack for RD)

Liquid from pear can
Lettuce or spinach leaves
Mayonnaise (low-calorie mayonnaise for RD)

Drain the liquid from pear can, and add enough water to make 1 cup. Bring to a gentle boil. Add gelatin and stir until dissolved. Chill until syrupy. Place each pear half in an individual mold, and cover with gelatin mixture. Chill until set. Unmold onto lettuce or spinach leaves. Garnish each portion with a dab of mayonnaise. Makes 4 servings.

Variation: Substitute canned peach halves for the pears.

Soup: An E/C Diet Support Food

SPRING SOUP

1 large head bibb or Boston
    lettuce
2 cups sorrel or spinach,
    coarsely chopped
2 stalks celery, diced
6 scallions, chopped
1½ quarts chicken stock
Salt and pepper to taste

2 tablespoons butter (FD) or
    dietetic margarine (RD)
2 teaspoons chopped fresh
    chervil
Sour cream (FD) or imitation
    sour cream (RD)
Lemon juice

Tear the lettuce leaves into small pieces, and combine with sorrel or spinach in a large saucepan. Add the celery, scallions, stock, salt, pepper, and butter or margarine. Cook over medium heat for 30 minutes, stirring occasionally. Remove from heat and sprinkle with chervil. Top each serving with a spoonful of sour cream, and sprinkle with a few drops of lemon juice. Makes 6 servings.

CHINESE CABBAGE SOUP WITH MEATBALLS

1 pound ground round
2 scallions, minced
½ teaspoon peanut oil
Soy sauce
Grated fresh ginger root
Pinch of dry mustard

7 cups beef stock or broth
1 large Chinese cabbage, cut in
    2-inch pieces
½ cup canned tomatoes
Chopped fresh parsley

Combine ground round, scallions, oil, and dry mustard. Add soy sauce and grated ginger root to taste. Shape into tiny meatballs.

Bring stock or broth to boil in a kettle. Drop in the meatballs, one at a time. Simmer over low heat until meatballs are cooked. Remove them to soup tureen and keep warm. Add cabbage and tomatoes to the soup. Cover and simmer until the cabbage is tender but still crisp—about 5 minutes. Ladle the soup over the meatballs. Sprinkle with chopped parsley. Makes 8 servings.

ANDALUSIAN COLD VEGETABLE SOUP

2 cucumbers, peeled, seeded, and chopped fine
1 tomato, peeled, seeded, and chopped fine
½ cup minced green pepper
½ cup minced Bermuda onion
3 hard-cooked eggs
1 tablespoon olive oil
1 clove garlic, crushed
1 teaspoon dry mustard

1 teaspoon Worcestershire sauce
6 cups tomato or V-8 vegetable juice
Juice of 1 lemon or lime
Tabasco
Salt and pepper
Sugar
Celery salt
Thin lemon slices
Chopped fresh parsley

In a large glass bowl, mash hard-cooked egg yolks with the olive oil to a smooth paste. (Reserve egg whites for garnish.) Blend in garlic, dry mustard, and Worcestershire sauce. Add cucumbers, tomato, green pepper, and onion. Combine tomato or vegetable juice with the lemon or lime juice. Pour over the vegetables. Season to taste with salt and pepper, a dash of Tabasco, a pinch of sugar and celery salt. Chill until icy cold. Serve with an ice cube or two in each bowl. Garnish with slivers of the reserved hard-cooked egg whites, lemon slices, and chopped parsley. Makes 6 servings.

CONSOMMÉ

3 pounds lean beef, cut in 1-inch cubes
2 pounds marrow bones
2 pounds veal knuckle
Chicken feet, giblets, wings, and bones
½ cup diced carrots
½ cup diced turnips
½ cup diced celery
½ cup diced onions

3 tablespoons butter (FD) or dietetic margarine (RD)
1 tablespoon salt
1½ teaspoons peppercorns
4 cloves
3 sprigs parsley
2 sprigs thyme
1 bay leaf
1 sprig marjoram

Brown half of the beef in half the marrow from marrow bones. Add remaining beef, marrow bones, veal knuckle, and 3½ quarts water. Bring slowly to a boil, then simmer for 3 hours, skimming off scum as it rises to the surface. Add chicken feet, giblets, wings, and bones along with another quart of water. Simmer for 2 more hours. Cook the vegetables in butter or margarine for about 6 minutes. Add to soup along with the seasonings and herbs. Continue simmering for another 1½ hours. Strain and skim off fat. Clear. Makes about 3 quarts.

Consommé with Celeriac: Heat consommé until piping hot. Serve in heated soup cups, and garnish each serving with thin slices of celeriac (celery root) which have been cooked until tender in salted water. Sprinkle with finely chopped fresh parsley.

Consommé with Herbs: Double the amount of herbs used in the recipe for consommé, and add 2 sprigs each of basil, rosemary, and chives.

Consommé Julienne: To each quart of consommé, add ½ cup cooked string beans, 1 sliced, cooked leek, and ¼ cup each of cooked carrots and turnips, cut in julienne strips.

Consommé with Mushrooms: Just before serving the hot consommé, add 1 tablespoon dry white wine and 2 or 3 sliced raw mushrooms to each serving.

TOMATO CONSOMMÉ

1 quart canned tomatoes
1 green pepper, seeded and chopped
2 stalks celery, sliced
1 carrot, sliced
1 small onion, sliced
4 cloves
¾ teaspoon peppercorns
Salt
Pepper

In a kettle, combine canned tomatoes, green pepper, celery, carrot, onion and seasonings with 1⅓ cups water. Bring to a boil, then simmer for 30 minutes. Season to taste with salt and pepper. Strain, cool, and clear. Serve piping hot. Makes 4 servings.

VENISON BROTH

4 pounds venison bones
1½ pounds scrap venison
4 stalks celery, with leaves, sliced
3 onions, finely chopped
3 carrots, finely chopped
1 clove garlic, minced
4 peppercorns
4 sprigs parsley
2 tomatoes, peeled and chopped
1 teaspoon juniper berries, snugly wrapped in muslin or cheesecloth
1 teaspoon salt
Thin lemon slices

Combine all the ingredients in a large soup kettle with 4 quarts of water. Bring to a boil. Lower heat, cover, and simmer for 2½ to 3 hours. Skim off the fat, and strain the soup through a very fine sieve. Chill. Remove the layer of fat on top, and reheat the soup. Garnish each portion with a thin lemon slice. Makes 8 servings.

BEEF AND TOMATO SOUP

4 cups beef bouillon
3 large, ripe tomatoes, peeled
  and chopped
½ pound ground shin of beef
1 leek, chopped

1 celery knob, chopped
Pinch of basil
2 beaten egg whites
Salt and pepper to taste
Chopped fresh parsley

Combine all the ingredients, except the chopped parsley, and simmer for 1 hour. Strain the soup through cheesecloth. Garnish with chopped fresh parsley. Makes 4 servings.

RED SNAPPER SOUP

2 pounds red snapper fillets
1 cup chopped tomatoes
½ cup tomato puree
¼ cup chopped green pepper
¼ cup chopped onion

2 tablespoons chopped celery
½ clove garlic, minced
Generous pinch of thyme
Salt and pepper

Cut fish into half-inch pieces. In a large saucepan, combine tomatoes, tomato puree, green pepper, onion, celery, garlic, and 5 cups of water. Bring to a boil. Then lower heat and simmer for about 30 minutes. Add fish and cook until it is tender. Beat the mixture with a wire whisk until the fish flakes. Add thyme and season to taste with salt and pepper. Makes 6 servings.

MINESTRONE

1 tablespoon butter (FD) or
  dietetic margarine (RD)
½ cup finely diced onions
½ cup finely diced celery
½ cup finely diced carrots
¼ cup finely diced green pepper
1 cup shredded cabbage
1 clove garlic, finely minced

1 teaspoon minced parsley
1 cup diced fresh tomatoes
4 beef bouillon cubes
½ cup elbow macaroni
1 cup chopped, young, tender
  spinach
Salt and pepper
Grated Parmesan cheese

Melt the butter or margarine in a large saucepan. Add onions, celery, carrots, green pepper, cabbage, garlic, and parsley. Cook over low heat for about 10 minutes, stirring frequently. Add tomatoes, 1 quart hot water, and bouillon cubes. Bring to a boil, then simmer until vegetables are tender. Meanwhile, cook the macaroni in boiling salted water until just tender. Drain and add to soup. Add chopped spinach and cook another 2 to 3 minutes. Season to taste with salt and pepper. Sprinkle with grated Parmesan cheese (1 tablespoon FD, 1 teaspoon RD). Makes 4 servings.

JELLIED BOUILLON

2 cups beef bouillon
1 cup chicken bouillon
1 cup tomato puree
2 egg whites, slightly beaten
2 crushed egg shells
1 onion, sliced

A few sprigs parsley
2 tablespoons gelatin
Salt and pepper to taste
Hard-cooked egg slices
Chopped fresh parsley or thin
 lemon slices

Combine the beef and chicken bouillon, tomato puree, egg whites, egg shells, onion, parsley, salt and pepper. Simmer for 12 to 15 minutes. Soak gelatin in a half cup cold water and add to soup. Let stand 10 minutes. Strain through a double thickness of cheesecloth. Place a hard-cooked egg slice at the bottom of each bouillon cup and fill with soup. Chill until firm. Garnish with chopped fresh parsley or a slice of lemon. Makes 6 servings.

SOPA CON ALBONDIGAS

(*Mexican Meat Ball Soup*)

¾ pound lean ground beef
1 egg, well beaten
¼ cup finely chopped onions
½ clove garlic, crushed
1 tablespoon minced parsley
1 teaspoon chili powder
½ teaspoon ground cumin

Salt and pepper to taste
Flour
6 cups beef bouillon
1 small bay leaf, crushed
1 cup canned tomatoes
1 egg, well beaten

Combine ground beef, egg, onions, garlic, parsley, chili powder, cumin, salt, and pepper. Mix well and shape into 1-inch balls. Dust with flour. Bring the bouillon to a boil, and drop in the meat balls. Cover and simmer slowly for 30 minutes. Add crushed bay leaf, tomatoes, and salt to taste. Cover and continue simmering for 30 minutes more. Gradually pour 1 cup of hot soup into the well beaten egg, stirring constantly. Return mixture to balance of soup and serve at once. Makes 6 servings.

BEET BORSCHT WITH YOGURT

1 No. 2 can shredded beets,
 undrained
4½ cups beef bouillon
6 tablespoons lemon juice
Few drops of onion juice

½ teaspoon salt
Pinch of pepper
Yogurt
Snipped dill

Combine beets, with their liquid, and bouillon in a large

saucepan. Bring to a boil, then simmer for 10 to 20 minutes. Add lemon juice and season with onion juice, salt, and pepper. Serve hot or chilled, each portion topped with a tablespoonful of yogurt and a sprinkling of snipped dill. Makes 6 servings.

JELLIED CUCUMBER SOUP

2 medium cucumbers, pared, seeded, and grated
1 small onion, grated
¼ cup finely chopped fresh mint leaves

6 cups jellied consommé, melted until syrupy
2 tablespoons lemon juice
Angostura bitters
Salt and white pepper

Combine the grated cucumbers and onion, mint leaves, and lemon juice. Stir into the consommé. Add a drop or two of bitters. Season to taste with salt and pepper. Spoon into soup cups and chill until set. Makes 6 to 8 servings.

CHINESE EGG-DROP SOUP

1 quart chicken broth or bouillon
⅛ teaspoon ground ginger
⅛ teaspoon Ac'cent
Soy sauce

3 eggs
2 tablespoons dry sherry
Sliced scallions (with green tops)

In a saucepan, combine broth or bouillon, ginger, and Ac'cent. Season to taste with soy sauce. Cover and bring to a boil. Lower heat. Meanwhile, beat the eggs with the sherry. Gradually drizzle egg mixture into the soup, stirring with a fork to separate egg into shreds. Sprinkle with sliced scallions. Serves 4 to 6.

CREAM OF WATERCRESS SOUP

1 bunch watercress
2 cups chicken stock or broth
2 tablespoons butter (FD) or dietetic margarine (RD)

2 tablespoons flour
2 cups milk
Salt
Pepper

Remove stems from watercress, and chop leaves very fine. Bring the stock or broth to a boil. Add watercress and simmer for 10 minutes. Melt the butter or margarine in another saucepan. Blend in the flour until smooth. Gradually stir in the milk and bring to a boil, stirring constantly. Simmer for 5 minutes. Combine the mixtures and season to taste with salt and pepper. Makes 4 servings.

COLD SUMMER SOUP

6 cups chilled tomato juice
1 small cucumber, thinly sliced
¼ cup chopped celery
3 scallions, finely chopped
Soy sauce
Lemon juice

Worcestershire sauce
Tabasco
Salt
Chopped fresh parsley or
    snipped dill

Combine tomato juice with cucumber, celery, and scallions. Season to taste with soy sauce, lemon juice, Worcestershire sauce, Tabasco, and salt. Garnish with chopped parsley or dill. Makes 6 servings.

CLAM AND TOMATO BROTH

Combine equal amounts of clam broth and tomato juice. Season to taste with Worcestershire sauce, lemon juice, and celery salt. Serve hot or chilled. Garnish each serving with a dollop of salted whipped cream (FD) or chopped fresh parsley (RD).

SCANDINAVIAN FISH SOUP

2 to 3 pounds haddock, cleaned
    but including bones, head,
    and tail
1 onion, sliced
1 carrot, sliced
2 stalks celery, with leaves,
    cut up
3 sprigs parsley
4 sprigs dill
1 bay leaf

3 cloves
1 slice of lemon
8 peppercorns
Salt to taste
2 tablespoons butter (FD) or
    dietetic margarine (RD)
2 tablespoons flour
2 cups milk (FD) or skimmed
    milk (RD)

Put the fish in soup kettle with 2 quarts of water. Add onion, carrot, celery, parsley, dill, bay leaf, lemon slice, cloves, peppercorns, and salt. Bring to a boil, then simmer for 45 minutes. Strain, reserving pieces of fish. In another pot, melt butter or margarine and blend in the flour. Gradually add the milk and stir until smooth. Add the broth and fish, and simmer for a few more minutes. Taste for seasoning. Makes 6 to 8 servings.

COLD SCHAV

1½ pounds schav (sorrel or
    sour grass), shredded
2 onions, minced, or 6 scallions,
    sliced
2 teaspoons salt
1 tablespoon lemon juice

4 tablespoons sugar (FD) or
    equivalent of artificial
    sweetener (RD)
2 eggs
Sour cream (imitation sour
    cream for RD)
Chopped hard-cooked egg

Combine the schav, onions, or scallions, and salt with two
quarts of water. Bring to a boil, then reduce flame and cook
over low heat for 45 minutes. Add the sugar or artificial
sweetener and lemon juice, and cook for an additional 15 minutes. Beat the eggs until lemon-colored. Gradually add a little
of the hot soup, stirring constantly to prevent curdling. Remove soup from heat and stir in the egg mixture. Chill thoroughly. Serve with a spoonful of sour cream in each portion.
Garnish with chopped hard-cooked egg. Makes 8 servings.

JAPANESE EGG SOUP

1½ quarts clear chicken
    bouillon
Soy sauce
Lemon juice
Ac'cent

12 snow peas
1 cucumber, sliced thin
6 eggs
Chopped scallions

Heat the bouillon, and season to taste with soy sauce, lemon
juice, and Ac'cent. Bring to a boil, then reduce heat. Add snow
peas and cucumber and simmer for 5 minutes. Transfer
vegetables to soup plates with a slotted spoon and keep warm.
Poach the eggs in the bouillon, and transfer one egg to each
soup plate. Strain the bouillon over the vegetables and eggs,
and sprinkle with chopped scallions. Makes 6 servings.

CHICKEN SOUP ORIENTALE

2 medium cucumbers, peeled,
    seeded, and chopped
¼ cup sliced celery
2 tablespoons butter (FD) or
    dietetic margarine (RD)
1½ quarts chicken stock

2 thin slices fresh ginger root,
    finely chopped
2 scallions, thinly sliced
1 tablespoon sherry
Soy sauce

Sauté cucumbers and celery in the butter or margarine for
about 1 minute. Add to the chicken stock along with the ginger

root, scallions, and sherry. Season to taste with soy sauce. Cover and simmer until piping hot. Makes 6 servings.

COTTAGE CHEESE SOUP

3 tablespoons butter (FD) or dietetic margarine (RD)
1 large onion, chopped
1 large green pepper, chopped
1 carrot, chopped
1 stalk celery, chopped
2 teaspoons minced parsley
½ teaspoon paprika
Salt and pepper to taste
3 cups milk (FD) or skimmed milk (RD)
2 cups cottage cheese
Snipped chives

Melt the butter or margarine in a large saucepan. Add the onion, green pepper, carrot, celery, and parsley, and cook for 15 minutes. Add paprika, salt, pepper, milk, and 3 cups of water. Cover and cook over low heat for one hour. Add the cottage cheese just before ready to serve. Heat, but do not let boil. Garnish with a sprinkling of snipped chives. Makes 8 servings.

PICKLE SOUP

5 dried mushrooms
2 quarts beef stock
2 onions, chopped
1 clove garlic, finely minced
1 carrot, sliced
1 stalk celery, sliced
1 bay leaf
3 small potatoes, peeled and diced
¼ pound cut string beans
Salt and pepper to taste
3 kosher-style pickles, diced
2 tablespoons chopped fresh parsley

Soak the mushrooms in water to cover for 1 hour. Drain well. Place them in a large saucepan with the beef stock, onions, garlic, carrot, celery, and bay leaf. Cover and simmer for about 45 minutes. Discard bay leaf, and put the mixture through a strainer. Return to saucepan and add potatoes, string beans, salt, pepper, and pickles. Cook over low heat until potatoes and string beans are done—about 15 minutes. If soup is too thick, add a little more beef stock. Add parsley and serve. Makes 8 servings.

BAVARIAN CHOWDER

¼ pound bologna, cut in
    ½-inch cubes
2 onions, chopped
½ green pepper, chopped
3 stalks celery, with leaves,
    finely sliced
2 small carrots, chopped
1 medium potato, diced

¼ head cabbage, shredded
1 cup canned tomatoes
1 cup beef bouillon
2 sprigs parsley
½ clove garlic
⅛ teaspoon thyme
Salt and pepper

Bring 3 cups of water to a boil and add the bologna. Simmer for 15 minutes. Add onions, green pepper, celery, carrots, potato, cabbage, tomatoes, beef bouillon, parsley, garlic and thyme. Season to taste with salt and pepper. Cover and simmer gently until all the vegetables are very tender—about 30 to 45 minutes. Makes 4 servings.

Appetite Snack Supports

THE OVERWEIGHT PERSON who has difficulty keeping to a diet suffers from an unruly appetite. The more stringent the diet, the more denied—the deeper the craving and the shorter the diet duration.

The overweight person eats for taste—and not hunger. So use the Appetite Supports to appease taste with tastily seasoned tidbits. A few calories in-between can reduce mealtime appetite. A *controlled* snack leads to a *controlled* appetite.

Use the foods listed judiciously to regulate your appetite.

Dill Pickles (excellent, mouth watering).

Pickling is good generally . . . and pickled vegetables such as cauliflower, pearl onions, and green tomatoes are fine lip-smackers. Pickling is a good idea for fish as well. Cook, cube, and refrigerate. Skewer with a toothpick for luscious morsels. Use halibut, bass, pike, etc. (No canned fish.)

Marinate small lamb cubes in lemon juice, pickling spices, garlic. Cook and refrigerate. Fix with sour-pickle tidbits for TV snack.

Do *something* with the list of garden greens below. Perhaps cooked with herbs and spices. Or crunchy, dipped gingerly in *boiled* salad dressing.

Carrots	Mushrooms
Celery	Radishes
Cucumber	Scallions
Green pepper	Tomatoes

The Energy-Controlled Malted Milk:

1 glass skim milk
4 strawberries
    or 1 teaspoon instant coffee
1 teaspoon artificial sweetener
3 ice cubes

Whirl in blender. It puffs up with lots of air and is *filling* as well as delicious!

Use spices to appease the taste buds. Even commonplace "allowed" foods make the juices flow when artfully seasoned. Use dill, basil, cinnamon, allspice, pepper, garlic salt, onion powder . . .

Small baked apples—prepared with No-Cal cherry soda, allspice or cinnamon, artificial sweetener to taste. Chill and reach for when the appetite threatens to cheat on the diet pattern. Use as an Appetite Support to save the (diet) day.

A tiny sweet. Two to four cream mints (half-inch cubes). The taste *lingers* . . .

For a delicacy, try a teaspoon of caviar on soda cracker. A little goes a long way. The taste is intense, and small nibbles at the "needing time" satisfy.

A green olive popped into the mouth as the eye begins to scan the horizon for potato chips, nuts, and buttered popcorn can divert catastrophe. One chip leads to another. But a few olives (up to four), with the pit long-lingering for each, can be a fine appetite control if reached for when a delectable food commercial comes on TV.

If sweets are your preference, the low-calorie sodas provide a tantalizing variety of fruit flavors. And the same goes for dietetic Jell-O!

And if sauerkraut is to your liking, go to it!

What People Weigh Now

NEW TABLE

OF AVERAGE WEIGHTS

	Height With Shoes	*Weight in Pounds in Indoor Clothing* Ages				
		20-24	25-29	30-39	40-49	50-59
MEN	5' 2"	128	134	137	140	142
	4"	136	141	145	148	149
	6"	142	148	153	156	157
	8"	149	155	161	165	166
	10"	157	163	170	174	175
	6' 0"	166	172	179	183	185
	2"	174	182	188	192	194
	4"	181	190	199	203	205
WOMEN	5' 0"	108	113	120	127	130
	2"	115	119	126	133	136
	4"	121	125	132	140	144
	6"	129	133	139	147	152
	8"	136	140	146	155	160
	10"	144	148	154	164	169
	6' 0"	154	158	164	174	180

Between ages 25 and 40, the average man gains 11 pounds.

The new average weights for men are about *5 pounds higher* than the earlier averages. In contrast, average weights of women under 40 have *decreased* about 3 pounds.

WEIGHT SCALE

What Is the "Best" Weight?

DESIRABLE WEIGHTS ACCORDING TO FRAME AT AGES 25 AND OVER

	Height With Shoes	Weight in Pounds in Indoor Clothing		
		Small Frame	Medium Frame	Large Frame
MEN	5' 2"	112-120	118-129	126-141
	4"	118-126	124-136	132-148
	6"	124-133	130-143	138-156
	8"	132-141	138-152	147-166
	10"	140-150	146-160	155-174
	6' 0"	148-158	154-170	164-184
	2"	156-167	162-180	173-194
	4"	164-175	172-190	182-204
WOMEN	5' 0"	96-104	101-113	109-125
	2"	102-110	107-119	115-131
	4"	108-116	113-126	121-138
	6"	114-123	120-135	129-146
	8"	122-131	128-143	137-154
	10"	130-140	136-151	145-163
	6' 0"	138-148	144-159	153-173

Computed by Metropolitan Life Insurance Company.

Other SIGNET Books of Interest